POWER THROUGH REPOSE

BY

ANNIE PAYSON CALL

Personality   binds—universality   expands.
FRANCOISE DELSARTE.

When the body is perfectly adjusted, perfectly supplied with force, perfectly free and works with the greatest economy of expenditure, it is fitted to be a perfect instrument alike of impression, experience, and expression.

W. R. ALGER.

CONTENTS

I.

THE GUIDANCE OF THE BODY

THE literature relating to the care of the human body is already very extensive. Much has been written about the body's proper food, the air it should breathe, the clothing by which it should be protected, the best methods of its development. That literature needs but little added to it, until we, as rational beings, come nearer to obeying the laws which it discloses, and to feeling daily the help which comes from that obedience.

It is of the better use, the truer guidance of this machine, that I wish especially to write. Although attention is constantly called to the fact of its misuse,—as in neglected rest and in over-strain,—in all the unlimited variety which the perverted ingenuity of a clever people has devised, it seems never to have come to any one's mind that this strain in all things, small and great, is something that can be and should be studiously abandoned, with as regular a process of training, from the first simple steps to those more complex, as is required in the work for the development of muscular strength. When a perversion of Nature's laws has continued from generation to generation, we, of the ninth or tenth generation, can by no possibility jump back into the place where the laws can work normally through us, even though our eyes have been opened to a full recognition of such perversion. We must climb back to an orderly life, step by step, and the compensation is large in the constantly growing realization of the greatness of the laws we have been disobeying. The appreciation of the power of a natural law, as it works through us, is one of the keenest pleasures that can come to man in this life.

The general impression seems to be that common-sense should lead us to a better use of our machines at once. Whereas, common-sense will not bring a true power of guiding the muscles, any more than it will cause the muscles' development, unless having the common-sense to see the need, we realize with it the necessity for cutting a path and walking in it. For the muscles' development, several paths have been cut, and many who are in need are walking in them, but, to the average man, the road to the best kind of muscular development still remains closed. The only training now in use is followed by sleight-of-hand performers, acrobats, or other jugglers, and that is limited to the professional needs of its followers.

Again, as the muscles are guided by means of the nerves, a training for the guidance of the muscles means, so far as the physique is concerned, first, a training for the better use of the nervous force. The nervous system is so wonderful in its present power for good or ill, so wonderful in its possible power either way, and so much more wonderful as we realize what we do not know about it, that it is not surprising that it is looked upon with awe. Neither is it strange that it seems to many, especially the ignorant, a subject to be shunned. It is not uncommon for a mother, whose daughter is suffering, and may be on the verge of nervous prostration because of her misused nerves, to say, "I do not want my daughter to know that she has nerves." The poor child knows it already in the wrong way. It is certainly better that she should know her nerves by learning a wholesome, natural use of them. The mother's remark is common with many men and women when speaking of themselves,—common with teachers when talking to or of their pupils. It is of course quite natural that it should be a prevailing idea, because hitherto the mention of nerves by man or woman has generally meant perverted nerves, and to dwell on our perversions, except long enough to shun them, is certainly unwholesome in the extreme.

II.

PERVERSIONS IN THE GUIDANCE OF THE BODY

SO evident are the various, the numberless perversions of our powers in the misuse of the machine, that it seems almost unnecessary to write of them. And yet, from another point of view, it is very necessary; for superabundant as they are, thrusting their evil results upon us every day in painful ways, still we have eyes and see not, ears and hear not, and for want of a fuller realization of these most grievous mistakes, we are in danger of plunging more and more deeply into the snarls to which they bring us. From nervous prostration to melancholia, or other forms of insanity, is not so long a step.

It is of course a natural sequence that the decadence of an entire country must follow the waning powers of the individual citizens. Although that seems very much to hint, it cannot be too much when we consider even briefly the results that have already come to us through this very misuse of our own voluntary powers. The advertisements of nerve medicines alone speak loudly to one who studies in the least degree the physical tendencies of the nation. Nothing proves better the artificial state of man, than the artificial means he uses to try to adjust himself to Nature's laws,—means which, in most cases, serve to assist him to keep up a little longer the appearance of natural life. For any simulation of that which is natural must sooner or later lead to nothing, or worse than nothing. Even the rest-cures, the most simple and harmless of the nerve restorers, serve a mistaken end. Patients go with nerves tired and worn out with misuse,—commonly called over-work. Through rest, Nature, with the warm, motherly help she is ever ready to bring us, restores the worn body to a normal state; but its owner has not learned to work the machine any better,—to drive his horses more naturally, or with a gentler hand. He knows he must take life more easily, but even with a passably good realization of that necessity, he can practise it only to a certain extent; and most occupants of rest-cures find themselves driven back more than once for another "rest."

Nervous disorders, resulting from overwork are all about us. Extreme nervous prostration is most prevalent. A thoughtful study of the faces around us, and a better understanding of their lives, brings to light many who are living, one might almost say, in a chronic state of nervous prostration, which lasts for years before the break comes. And because of the want of thought, the want of study for a better, more natural use of the machine, few of us appreciate our own possible powers. When with study the appreciation grows, it is a daily surprise, a constantly increasing delight.

Extreme nervous tension seems to be so peculiarly American, that a German physician coming to this country to practise became puzzled by the variety of nervous disorders he was called upon to help, and finally announced his discovery of a new disease which he chose to call "Americanitis." And now we suffer from "Americanitis" in all its unlimited varieties. Doctors study it; nerve medicines arise on every side; nervine hospitals establish themselves; and rest-cures innumerable spring up in all directions,—but the root of the matter is so comparatively simple that in general it is overlooked entirely.

When illnesses are caused by disobedience to the perfect laws of Nature, a steady, careful obedience to these laws will bring us to a healthful state again.

Nature is so wonderfully kind that if we go one-tenth of the way, she will help us the other nine-tenths. Indeed she seems to be watching and hoping for a place to get in, so quickly does she take possession of us, if we do but turn toward her ever so little. But instead of adopting her simple laws and following quietly her perfect way, we try by every artificial means to gain a rapid transit back to her dominion, and succeed only in getting farther away from her. Where is the use of taking medicines to give us new strength, while at the same time we are steadily disobeying the very laws from the observance of which alone the strength can come? No medicine can work in a man's-body while the man's habits are constantly counteracting it. More harm than good is done in the end. Where is the use of all the quieting medicines, if we only quiet our nerves in order that we may continue to misuse them without their crying out? They will cry out sooner or later; for Nature, who is so quick to help us to the true way of living, loses patience at last, and her punishments are justly severe. Or, we might better say, a law is fixed and immovable, and if we disobey and continue to disobey it, we suffer the consequences.

III.

REST IN SLEEP

HOW do we misuse our nervous force? First, let us consider, When should the body be completely at rest? The longest and most perfect rest should be during sleep at night. In sleep we can accomplish nothing in the way of voluntary activity either of mind or body. Any nervous or muscular effort during sleep is not only useless but worse,—it is pure waste of fuel, and results in direct and irreparable harm. Realizing fully that sleep is meant for rest, that the only gain is rest, and that new power for use comes as a consequence,—how absurd it seems that we do not abandon ourselves completely to gaining all that Nature would give us through sleep.

Suppose, instead of eating our dinner, we should throw the food out of the window, give it to the dogs, do anything with it but what Nature meant we should, and then wonder why we were not nourished, and why we suffered from faintness and want of strength. It would be no more senseless than the way in which most of us try to sleep now, and then wonder why we are not better rested from eight hours in bed. Only this matter of fatiguing sleep has crept upon us so slowly that we are blind to it. We disobey mechanically all the laws of Nature in sleep, simple as they are, and are so blinded by our own immediate and personal interests, that the habit of not resting when we sleep has grown to such an extent that to return to natural sleep, we must think, study, and practise.

Few who pretend to rest give up entirely to the bed, a dead weight,—letting the bed hold them, instead of trying to hold themselves on the bed. Watch, and unless you are an exceptional case (of which happily there are a few), you will be surprised to see how you are holding yourself on the bed, with tense muscles, if not all over, so nearly all over that a little more tension would hardly increase the fatigue with which you are working yourself to sleep.

The spine seems to be the central point of tension—it does not *give* to the bed and rest there easily from end to end; it touches at each end and just so far along from each end as the man or woman who is holding it will permit. The knees are drawn up, the muscles of the legs tense, the hands and arms contracted, and the fingers clinched, either holding the pillow or themselves.

The head, instead of letting the pillow have its full weight, holds itself onto the pillow. The tongue cleaves to the roof of the mouth, the throat muscles are contracted, and the muscles of the face drawn up in one way or another.

This seems like a list of horrors, somewhat exaggerated when we realize that it is of sleep, "Tired Nature's sweet restorer," that we are speaking; but indeed it is only too true.

Of course cases are not in the majority where the being supposed to enjoy repose is using *all* these numerous possibilities of contraction. But there are very few who have not, unconsciously, some one or two or half-dozen nervous and muscular strains; and even after they become conscious of the useless contractions, it takes time and watchfulness and patience to relax out of them, the habit so grows upon us. One would think that even though we go to sleep in a tense way, after being once soundly off Nature could gain the advantage over us, and relax the muscles in spite of ourselves; but the habits of inheritance and of years are too much for her. Although she is so constantly gracious and kind, she cannot go out of her way, and we cannot ask her to do so.

How simple it seems to sleep in the right way; and how wholesome it is even to think about it, in contrast to the wrong way into which so many of us have fallen. If we once see clearly the great compensation in getting back to the only way of gaining restful sleep, the process is very simple, although because we were so far out of the right path it often seems slow. But once gained, or even partially gained, one great enemy to healthful, natural nerves is conquered, and has no possibility of power.

Of course the mind and its rapid and misdirected working is a strong preventive of free nerves, relaxed muscles, and natural sleep. "If I could only stop myself from thinking" is a complaint often heard, and reason or philosophy does not seem to touch it. Even the certain knowledge that nothing is gained by this rapid thought at the wrong time, that very much is lost, makes no impression on the overwrought mind,—often even excites it more, which proves that the trouble, if originally mental, has now gained such a hold upon the physique that it must be attacked there first. The nerves should be trained to enable the body to be an obedient servant to a healthy mind, and the mind in giving its attention to such training gains in normal power of direction.

If you cannot stop thinking, do not try; let your thoughts steam ahead if they will. Only relax your muscles, and as the attention is more and more fixed on the interesting process of letting-go of the muscles (interesting, simply because the end is so well worth gaining), the imps of thought find less and less to take hold of, and the machinery in the head must stop its senseless working, because the mind which allowed it to work has applied itself to something worth accomplishing.

The body should also be at rest in necessary reclining in the day, where of course all the laws of sleep apply. Five minutes of complete rest in that way means greater gain than an hour or three hours taken in the usual manner. I remember watching a woman "resting" on a lounge, propped up with the downiest of pillows, holding her head perfectly erect and in a strained position, when it not only would have been easier to let it fall back on the pillow, but it seemed impossible that she should not let it go; and yet there it was, held erect with an evident strain. Hers is not an unusual case, on the contrary quite a common one. Can we wonder that the German doctor thought he had discovered a new disease? And must he not be already surprised and shocked at the precocious growth of the infant monster which he found and named? "So prone are mortals to their own damnation, it seems as though a devil's use were gone."

There is no better way of learning to overcome these perversions in sleep and similar forms of rest, than to study with careful thought the sleep of a wholesome little child. Having gained the physical freedom necessary to give perfect repose to the body, the quiet, simple dropping of all thought and care can be made more easily possible. So we can approach again the natural sleep and enjoy consciously the refreshment which through our own babyhood was the unconscious means of giving us daily strength and power for growth.

To take the regular process, first let go of the muscles,—that will enable us more easily to drop disturbing thoughts; and as we refuse, without resistance, admittance to the thoughts, the freedom from care for the time will follow, and the rest gained will enable us to awaken with new life for cares to come. This, however, is a habit to be established and thoughtfully cultivated; it cannot be acquired at once. More will be said in future chapters as to the process of gaining the habit.

IV.

OTHER FORMS OF REST

DO you hold yourself on the chair, or does the chair hold you? When you are subject to the laws of gravitation give up to them, and feel their strength. Do not resist these laws, as a thousand and one of us do when instead of yielding gently and letting ourselves sink into a chair, we *put* our bodies rigidly on and then hold them there as if fearing the chair would break if we gave our full weight to it. It is not only unnatural and unrestful, but most awkward. So in a railroad car. Much, indeed most of the fatigue from a long journey by rail is quite unnecessary, and comes from an unconscious officious effort of trying to carry the train, instead of allowing the train to carry us, or of resisting the motion, instead of relaxing and yielding to it. There is a pleasant rhythm in the motion of the rapidly moving cars which is often restful rather than fatiguing, if we will only let go and abandon ourselves to it. This was strikingly proved by a woman who, having just learned the first principles of relaxation, started on a journey overstrained from mental anxiety. The first effect of the motion was that most disagreeable, faint feeling known as car-sickness. Understanding the cause, she began at once to drop the unnecessary tension, and the faintness left her. Then she commenced an interesting novel, and as she became excited by the plot her muscles were contracted in sympathy (so-called), and the faintness returned in full force, so that she had to drop the book and relax again; and this process was repeated half-a-dozen times before she could place her body so under control of natural laws that it was possible to read without the artificial tension asserting itself and the car-sickness returning in consequence.

The same law is illustrated in driving. "I cannot drive, it tires me so," is a common complaint. Why does it tire you? Because instead of yielding entirely and freely to the seat of the carriage first, and then to its motion, you try to help the horses, or to hold yourself still while the carriage is moving. A man should become one with a carriage in driving, as much as one with his horse in riding. Notice the condition in any place where there is excuse for some anxiety,—while going rather sharply round a corner, or nearing a railroad track. If your feet are not pressed forcibly against the floor of the carriage, the tension will be somewhere else. You are using nervous force to no earthly purpose, and to great earthly loss. Where any tension is necessary to make things better, it will assert itself naturally and more truly as we learn to drop all useless and harmful tension. Take a patient suffering from nervous prostration for a long drive, and you will bring him back more nervously prostrated; even the fresh air will not counteract the strain that comes from not knowing how to relax to the motion of the carriage.

A large amount of nervous energy is expended unnecessarily while waiting. If we are obliged to wait for any length of time, it does not hurry the minutes or bring that for which we wait to keep nervously strained with impatience; and it does use vital force, and so helps greatly toward "Americanitis." The strain which comes from an hour's nervous waiting, when simply to let yourself alone and keep still would answer much better, is often equal to a day's labor. It must be left to individuals to discover how this applies in their own especial cases, and it will be surprising to see not only how great and how common such strain is, but how comparatively easy it is to drop it. There are of course exceptional times and states when only constant trying and thoughtful watchfulness will bring any marked result.

We have taken a few examples where there is nothing to do but keep quiet, body and brain, from what should be the absolute rest of sleep to the enforced rest of waiting. Just one word more in connection with waiting and driving. You must catch a certain train. Not having time to trust to your legs or the cars, you hastily take a cab. You will in your anxiety keep up exactly the same strain that you would have had in walking,—as if you could help the carriage along, or as if reaching the station in time depended upon your keeping a rigid spine and tense muscles. You have hired the carriage to take you, and any activity on your part is quite unnecessary until you reach the station; why not keep quiet and let the horses do the work, and the driver attend to his business?

It would be easy to fill a small volume with examples of the way in which we are walking directly into nervous prostration; examples only of this one variety of disobedience,—namely, of the laws of *rest*. And to give illustrations of all the varieties of disobedience to Nature's laws in *activity* would fill not one small book, but several large ones; and then, unless we improve, a year-book of new examples of nervous strain could be published. But fortunately, if we are nervous and short-sighted, we have a good share of brain and commonsense when it is once appealed to, and a few examples will open our eyes and set us thinking, to real and practical results.

V.

THE USE OF THE BRAIN

LET us now consider instances where the brain alone is used, and the other parts of the body have nothing to do but keep quiet and let the brain do its work. Take thinking, for instance. Most of us think with the throat so contracted that it is surprising there is room enough to let the breath through, the tongue held firmly, and the jaw muscles set as if suffering from an acute attack of lockjaw. Each has his own favorite tension in the act of meditation, although we are most generous in the force given to the jaw and throat. The same superfluous tension may be observed in one engaged in silent reading; and the force of the strain increases in proportion to the interest or profundity of the matter read. It is certainly clear, without a knowledge of anatomy or physiology, that for pure, unadulterated thinking, only the brain is needed; and if vital force is given to other parts of the body to hold them in unnatural contraction; we not only expend it extravagantly, but we rob the brain of its own. When, for purely mental work, all the activity is given to the brain, and the body left free and passive, the concentration is better, conclusions are reached

14

with more satisfaction, and the reaction, after the work is over, is healthy and refreshing.

This whole machine can be understood perhaps more clearly by comparing it to a community of people. In any community,—Church, State, institution, or household,—just so far as each member minds his own business, does his own individual work for himself and for those about him, and does not officiously interfere with the business of others, the community is quiet, orderly, and successful. Imagine the state of a deliberative assembly during the delivery of a speech, if half-a-dozen of the listeners were to attempt to help the speaker by rising and talking at the same time; and yet this is the absurd action of the human body when a dozen or more parts, that are not needed, contract "in sympathy" with those that have the work to do. It is an unnecessary brace that means loss of power and useless fatigue. One would think that the human machine having only one mind, and the community many thousands, the former would be in a more orderly state than the latter.

In listening attentively, only the brain and ears are needed; but watch the individuals at an entertaining lecture, or in church with a stirring preacher. They are listening with their spines, their shoulders, the muscles of their faces. I do not refer to the look of interest and attention, or to any of the various expressions which are the natural and true reflection of the state of the mind, but to the strained attention which draws the facial muscles, not at all in sympathy with the speaker, but as a consequence of the tense nerves and contracted muscles of the listener. "I do not understand why I have this peculiar sort of asthma every Sunday afternoon," a lady said to me. She was in the habit of hearing, Sunday morning, a preacher, exceedingly interesting, but with a very rapid utterance, and whose mind travelled so fast that the words embodying his thoughts often tumbled over one another. She listened with all her nerves, as well as with those needed, held her breath when he stumbled, to assist him in finding his verbal legs, reflected every action with twice the force the preacher himself gave,—and then wondered why on Sunday afternoon, and at no other time, she had this nervous catching of the breath. She saw as soon as her attention was drawn to the general principles of Nature, how she had disobeyed this one, and why she had trouble on Sunday afternoon. This case is very amusing, even laughable, but it is a fair example of many similar nervous attacks, greater or less; and how easy it is to see that a whole series of these, day after day, doing their work unconsciously to the victim, will sooner or later bring some form of nervous prostration.

The same attitudes and the same effects often attend listening to music. It is a common experience to be completely fagged after two hours of delightful music. There is no exaggeration in saying that we should be *rested* after a good concert, if it is not too long. And yet so upside-down are we in our ways of living, and, through the mistakes of our ancestors, so accustomed have we become to disobeying Nature's laws, that the general impression seems to be that music cannot be fully enjoyed without a strained attitude of mind and body; whereas, in reality, it is much more exquisitely appreciated and enjoyed in Nature's way. If the nerves are perfectly free, they will catch the rhythm of the music, and so be helped back to the true rhythm of Nature, they will respond to the harmony and melody with all the vibratory power that God gave them, and how can the result be anything else than rest and refreshment,—unless having allowed them to vibrate in one direction too long, we have disobeyed a law in another way.

Our bodies cannot by any possibility be *free,* so long as they are strained by our own personal effort. So long as our nervous force is misdirected in personal strain, we can no more give full and responsive attention to the music, than a piano can sound the harmonies of a sonata if some one is drawing his hands at the same time backwards and forwards over the strings. But, alas! a contracted personality is so much the order of the day that many of us carry the chronic contractions of years constantly with us, and can no more free ourselves for a concert at a day's or a week's notice, than we can gain freedom to receive all the grand universal truths that are so steadily helpful. It is only by daily patience and thought and care that we can cease to be an obstruction to the best power for giving and receiving.

There are, scattered here and there, people who have not lost the natural way of listening to music,—people who are musicians through and through so that the moment they hear a fine strain they are one with it. Singularly enough the majority of these are fine animals, most perfectly and normally developed in their senses. When the intellect begins to assert itself to any extent, then the nervous strain comes. So noticeable is this, in many cases, that nervous excitement seems often to be from misdirected intellect; and people under the control of their misdirected nervous force often appear wanting in quick intellectual power,—

illustrating the law that a stream spreading in all directions over a meadow loses the force that the same amount of water would have if concentrated and flowing in one channel. There are also many cases where the strained nerves bring an abnormal intellectual action. Fortunately for the saving of the nation, there are people who from a physical standpoint live naturally. These are refreshing to see; but they are apt to take life too easily, to have no right care or thought, and to be sublimely selfish.

Another way in which the brain is constantly used is through the eyes. What deadly fatigue comes from time spent in picture galleries! There the strain is necessarily greater than in listening, because all the pictures and all the colors are before us at once, with no appreciable interval between forms and subjects that differ widely. But as the strain is greater, so should the care to relieve it increase. We should not go out too far to meet the pictures, but be quiet, and let the pictures come to us. The fatigue can be prevented if we know when to stop, and pleasure at the time and in the memory afterwards will be surprisingly increased. So is it in watching a landscape from the car window, and in all interests which come from looking. I am not for one instant condemning the *natural* expression of pleasure, neither do I mean that there should be any apparent nonchalance or want of interest; on the contrary, the real interest and its true expression increase as we learn to shun the shams.

But will not the discovery of all this superfluous tension make one self-conscious? Certainly it will for a time, and it must do so. You must be conscious of a smooch on your face in order to wash it off, and when the face is clean you think no more of it. So you must see an evil before you can shun it. All these physical evils you must be vividly conscious of, and when you are so annoyed as to feel the necessity of moving from under them self-consciousness decreases in equal ratio with the success of your efforts.

Whenever the brain alone is used in thinking, or in receiving and taking note of impressions through either of the senses, new power comes as we gain freedom from all misdirected force, and with muscles in repose leave the brain to quietly do its work without useless strain of any kind. It is of course evident that this freedom cannot be gained without, first, a consciousness of its necessity. The perfect freedom, however, when reached, means freedom from self-consciousness as well as from the strain which made self-consciousness for a time essential.

VI.

THE BRAIN IN ITS DIRECTION OF THE BODY

WE come now to the brain and its direction of other parts of the body.

What tremendous and unnecessary force is used in talking,—from the aimless motion of the hands, the shoulders, the feet, the entire body, to a certain rigidity of carriage, which tells as powerfully in the wear and tear of the nervous system as superfluous motion. It is a curious discovery when we find often how we are holding our shoulders in place, and in the wrong place. A woman receiving a visitor not only talks all over herself, but reflects the visitor's talking all over, and so at the end of the visit is doubly fatigued. "It tires me so to see people" is heard often, not only from those who are under the full influence of "Americanitis," but from many who are simply hovering about its borders. "Of course it tires you to see people, you see them with, so much superfluous effort," can almost without exception be a true answer. A very little simple teaching will free a woman from that unnecessary fatigue. If she is sensible, once having had her attention brought and made keenly alive to the fact that she talks all over, she will through constant correction gain the power of talking as Nature meant she should, with her vocal apparatus only, and with such easy motions as may be needed to illustrate her words. In this change, so far from losing animation, she gains it, and gains true expressive power; for all unnecessary motion of the body in talking simply raises a dust, so to speak, and really blurs the true thought of the mind and feeling of the heart.

The American voice—especially the female voice—is a target which has been hit hard many times, and very justly. A ladies' luncheon can often be truly and aptly compared to a poultry-yard, the shrill cackle being even more unpleasant than that of a large concourse of hens. If we had once become truly appreciative of the natural mellow tones possible to every woman, these shrill voices would no more be tolerated than a fashionable luncheon would be served in the kitchen.

A beautiful voice has been compared to corn, oil, and wine. We lack almost entirely the corn and the oil; and the wine in our voices is far more inclined to the sharp, unpleasant taste of very poor currant wine, than to the rich, spicy flavor of fine wine from the grape. It is not in the province of this book to consider the physiology of the voice, which would be necessary in order to show clearly how its natural laws are constantly disobeyed. We can now speak of it only with regard to the tension which is the immediate cause of the trouble. The effort to propel the voice from the throat, and use force in those most delicate muscles when it should come from the stronger muscles of the diaphragm, is like trying to make one man do the work of ten; the result must eventually be the utter collapse of the one man from over-activity, and loss of power in the ten men because of muscles unused. Clergyman's sore throat is almost always explainable in this way; and there are many laymen with constant trouble in the throat from no cause except the misuse of its muscles in talking. "The old philosopher said the seat of the soul was in the diaphragm. However that may be, the word begins there, soul and body; but you squeeze the life out of it in your throat, and so your words are born dead!" was the most expressive exclamation of an able trainer of the voice.

Few of us feel that we can take the time or exercise the care for the proper training of our voices; and such training is not made a prominent feature, as it should be, in all American schools. Indeed, if it were, we would have to begin with the teachers; for the typical teacher's voice, especially in our public schools, coming from unnecessary nervous strain is something frightful. In a large school-room a teacher can be heard, and more impressively heard, in common conversational tones; for then it is her mind that is felt more than her body. But the teacher's voice mounts the scale of shrillness and force just in proportion as her nervous fatigue increases; and often a true enthusiasm expresses itself—or, more correctly, hides itself—in a sharp, loud voice, when it would be far more effective in its power with the pupils if the voice were kept quiet. If we cannot give time or money to the best development of our voices, we can grow sensitive to the shrill, unpleasant tones, and by a constant preaching of "lower your voices," "speak more quietly," from the teacher to herself, and then to her pupils, from mother to child, and from every woman to her own voice, the standard American voice would change, greatly to the national advantage.

I never shall forget the restful pleasure of hearing a teacher call the roll in a large schoolroom as quietly as she would speak to a child in a closet, and every girl answering in the same soft and pleasant way. The effect even of that daily roll-call could not have been small in its counteracting influence on the shrill American tone.

Watch two people in an argument, as the excitement increases the voice rises. In such a case one of the best and surest ways to govern your temper is to lower your voice. Indeed the nervous system and the voice are in such exquisite sympathy that they constantly act and react on each other. It is always easier to relax superfluous tension after lowering the voice.

"Take the bone and flesh sound from your voice" is a simple and interesting direction. It means do not push so hard with your body and so interfere with the expression of your soul. Thumping on a piano, or hard scraping on a violin, will keep all possible expression from the music, and in just the same proportion will unnecessary physical force hide the soul in a voice. Indeed with the voice—because the instrument is finer—the contrast between Nature's way and man's perversion is far greater.

One of the first cares with a nervous invalid, or with any one who suffers at all from overstrained nerves, should be for a quiet, mellow voice. It is not an invariable truth that women with poorly balanced nerves have shrill, strained voices. There is also a rigid tone in a nervously low voice, which, though not unpleasant to the general ear, is expressive to one who is in the habit of noticing nervous people, and is much more difficult to relax than the high pitched voices. There is also a forced calm which is tremendous in its nervous strain, the more so as its owner takes pride in what she considers remarkable self-control.

Another common cause of fatigue with women is the useless strain in sewing. "I get so tired in the back of my neck" is a frequent complaint. "It is because you sew with the back of your neck" is generally the correct explanation. And it is because you sew with the muscles of your waist that they feel so strangely fatigued, and the same with the muscles of your legs or your chest. Wherever the tired feeling comes it is because of unnatural and officious tension, which, as soon as the woman becomes sensible of it, can be stopped entirely by taking two or three minutes now and then to let go of these wrongly sympathetic muscles and so teach them to mind their own business, and sew with only the muscles that are needed. A very simple cause of over-fatigue in sewing is the cramped, strained position of the lungs; this can be prevented without even stopping in the work, by taking long, quiet, easy breaths. Here there must be *no exertion whatever* in the chest muscles. The lungs must seem to expand from the pressure of the air alone, as independently as a rubber ball will expand when external pressure is removed, and they must be allowed to expel the air with the same independence. In this way the growth of breathing power will be slow, but it will be sure and delightfully restful. Frequent, full, quiet breaths might be the means of relief to many sufferers, if only they would take the trouble to practise them faithfully,—a very slight effort compared with the result which will surely ensue. And so it is with the fatigue from sewing. I fear I do not exaggerate, when I say that in nine cases out of ten a woman would rather sew with a pain in her neck than stop for the few moments it would take to relax it and teach it truer habits, so that in the end the pain might be avoided entirely. Then, when the inevitable nervous exhaustion follows, and all the kindred troubles that grow out of it she pities herself and is pitied by others, and wonders why God thought best to afflict her with suffering and illness. "Thought best!" God never thought best to give any one pain. He made His laws, and they are wholesome and perfect and true, and if we disobey them we must suffer the consequences! I knock my head hard against a stone and then wonder why God thought best to give me the headache. There would be as much sense in that as there is in much of the so-called Christian resignation to be found in the world to-day. To be sure there are inherited illnesses and pains, physical and mental, but the laws are so made that the compensation of clear-sightedness and power for use gained by working our way rightly out of all inheritances and suffering brought by others, fully equalizes any apparent loss.

In writing there is much unnecessary nervous fatigue. The same cramped attitude of the lungs that accompanies sewing can be counteracted in the same way, although in neither case should a cramped attitude be allowed at all Still the relief of a long breath is always helpful and even necessary where one must sit in one position for any length of time. Almost any even moderately nervous man or woman will hold a pen as if some unseen force were trying to pull it away, and will write with firmly set jaw, contracted throat, and a powerful tension in the muscles of the tongue, or whatever happens to be the most officious part of this especial individual community. To swing the pendulum to another extreme seems not to enter people's minds when trying to find a happy medium. Writer's paralysis, or even the ache that comes from holding the hand so long in a more or less cramped attitude, is easily obviated by stopping once in an hour or half hour, stretching the fingers wide and letting the muscles slowly relax of their own accord. Repeat this half-a-dozen times, and after each exercise try to hold the pen or pencil with natural lightness; it will not take many days to change the habit of tension to one of ease, although if you are a steady writer the stretching exercise will always be necessary, but much less often than at first.

In lifting a heavyweight, as in nursing the sick, the relief is immediate from all straining in the back, by pressing hard with the feet on the floor and *thinking* the power of lifting in the legs. There is true economy of nervous force here, and a sensitive spine is freed from a burden of strain which might undoubtedly be the origin of nervous prostration. I have made nurses practise lifting, while impressing the fact forcibly upon them by repetition before they lift, and during the process of raising a body and lowering it, that they must use entirely the muscles of the legs. When once their minds have full comprehension of the new way, the surprise with which they discover the comparative ease of lifting is very pleasant. The whole secret in this and all similar efforts is to use muscular instead of nervous force. Direct with the directing power; work with the working power.

VII.

THE DIRECTION OF THE BODY IN LOCOMOTION

LIFTING brings us to the use of the entire body, which is considered simply in the most common of all its movements,—that of walking.

The rhythm of a perfect walk is not only delightful, but restful; so that having once gained a natural walk there is no pleasanter way to rest from brain fatigue than by means of this muscle fatigue. And yet we are constantly contradicting and interfering with Nature in walking. Women—perhaps partly owing to their unfortunate style of dress—seem to hold themselves together as if fearing that having once given their muscles free play, they would fall to pieces entirely. Rather than move easily forward, and for fear they might tumble to pieces, they shake their shoulders and hips from side to side, hold their arms perfectly rigid from the shoulders down, and instead of the easy, natural swing that the motion of walking would give the arms, they go forward and back with no regularity, but are in a chronic state of jerk. The very force used in holding an arm as stiff as the ordinary woman holds it, would be enough to give her an extra mile in every five-mile walk. Then again, the muscles of the throat must help, and more than anywhere else is force unnecessarily expended in the waist muscles. They can be very soon felt, pushing with all their might—and it is not a small might—officiously trying to assist in the action of the legs; whereas if they would only let go, mind their own business, and let the legs swing easily as if from the shoulders, they might reflect the rhythmic motion, and gain in a true freedom and power. Of course all this waste of force comes from nervous strain and is nervous strain, and a long walk in the open air, when so much of the new life gained is wrongly expended, does not begin to do the good work that might be accomplished. To walk with your muscles and not use superfluous nervous force is the first thing to be learned, and after or at the same time to direct your muscles as Nature meant they should be directed,—indeed we might almost say to let Nature direct them herself, without our interference. Hurry with your muscles and not with your nerves. This tells especially in hurrying for a train, where the nervous anxiety in the fear of losing it wakes all possible unnecessary tension and often impedes the motion instead of assisting it. The same law applies here that was mentioned before with regard to the carriage,—only instead of being quiet and letting the carriage take you, be quiet and let your walking machine do its work. So in all hurrying, and the warning can hardly be given too many times, we must use our nerves only as transmitters—calm, well-balanced transmitters—that our muscles may be more efficient and more able servants.

The same mistakes of unnecessary tension will be found in running, and, indeed, in all bodily motion, where the machine is not trained to do its work with only the nerves and muscles needed for the purpose. We shall have opportunity to consider these motions in a new light when we come to the directions for gaining a power of natural motion; now we are dealing only with mistakes.

VIII.

NERVOUS STRAIN IN PAIN AND SICKNESS

THERE is no way in which superfluous and dangerous tension is so rapidly increased as in the bearing of pain. The general impression seems to be that one should brace up to a pain; and very great strength of will is often shown in the effort made and the success achieved in bearing severe pain by means of this bracing process. But alas, the reaction after the pain is over—that alone would show the very sad misuse which had been made of a strong will. Not that there need be no reaction; but it follows naturally that the more strain brought to bear upon the nervous system in endurance, the greater must be the reaction when the load is lifted. Indeed, so well is this known in the medical profession, that it is a surgical axiom that the patient who most completely controls his expression of pain will be the greatest sufferer from the subsequent reaction. While there is so much pain to be endured in this world, a study of how best to bear it certainly is not out of place, especially when decided practical effects can be quickly shown as the result of such study. So prevalent is the idea that a pain is better borne by clinching the fists and tightening all other muscles in the body correspondingly, that I know the possibility of a better or more natural mode of endurance will be laughed at by many, and others will say, "That is all very well for those who can relax to a pain,—let them gain from it, I cannot; it is natural for me to set my teeth and bear it." There is a distinct difference between what is natural to us and natural to Nature, although the first term is of course misused.

Pain comes from an abnormal state of some part of the nervous system. The more the nerves are strained to bear pain, the more sensitive they become; and of course those affected immediately feel most keenly the increased sensitiveness, and so the pain grows worse. Reverse that action, and through the force of our own inhibitory power let a new pain be a reminder to us to *let go,* instead of to hold on, and by decreasing the strain we decrease the possibility of more pain. Whatever reaction may follow pain then, will be reaction from the pain itself, not from the abnormal tension which has been held for the purpose of bearing it.

But—it will be objected—is not the very effort of the brain to relax the tension a nervous strain? Yes, it is,—not so great, however, as the continued tension all over the body, and it grows less and less as the habit is acquired of bearing the pain easily. The strain decreases more rapidly with those who having undertaken to relax, perceive the immediate effects; for, of course, as the path clears and new light comes they are encouraged to walk more steadily in the easier way.

I know there are pains that are better borne and even helped by a certain amount of *bracing,* but if the idea of bearing such pain quietly, easily, naturally, takes a strong hold of the mind, all bracing will be with a true equilibrium of the muscles, and will have the required effect without superfluous tension.

One of the most simple instances of bearing pain more easily by relaxing to it occurs while sitting in the dentist's chair. Most of us clutch the arms, push with our feet, and hold ourselves off the chair to the best of our ability. Every nerve is alive with the expectation of being hurt.

The fatigue which results from an hour or more of this dentist tension is too well known to need description. Most of the nervous fatigue suffered from the dentist's work is in consequence of the unnecessary strain of expecting a hurt and not from any actual pain inflicted. The result obtained by insisting upon making yourself a dead weight in the chair, if you succeed only partially, will prove this. It will also be a preliminary means of getting well rid of the dentist fright,—that peculiar dread which is so well known to most of us. The effect of fright is nervous strain, which again contracts the muscles. If we drop the muscular tension, and so the nervous strain, thus working our way into the cause by means of the effect, there will be no nerves or muscles to hold the fright, which then so far as the physique is concerned cannot exist. *So far as the physique is concerned,*—that is emphatic; for as we work inward from the effect to the cause we must be met by the true philosophy inside, to accomplish the whole work. I might relax my body out of the nervous strain of fright all day; if my mind insisted upon being frightened it would simply be a process of freeing my nerves and muscles that they might be made more effectually tense by an unbalanced, miserably controlled mind. In training to bring body and mind to a more normal state, the teacher must often begin with the body only, and use his own mind to gently lead the pupil to clearer sight. Then when the pupil can strike the equilibrium between mind and body,—he must be left to acquire the habit for himself.

The same principles by which bearing the work of the dentist is made easier, are applicable in all pain, and especially helpful when pain is nervously exaggerated. It would be useless and impossible to follow the list of various pains which we attempt to bear by means of additional strain.

Each of us has his own personal temptation in the way of pain,—from the dentist's chair to the most severe suffering, or the most painful operation,—and each can apply for himself the better way of bearing it. And it is not perhaps out of place here to speak of the taking of ether or any anaesthetic before an operation. The power of relaxing to the process easily and quietly brings a quicker and pleasanter effect with less disagreeable results. One must take ether easily in mind and body. It a man forces himself to be quiet externally, and is frightened and excited mentally, as soon as he has become unconscious enough to lose control of his voluntary muscles, the impression of fright made upon the brain asserts itself, and he struggles and resists in proportion.

These same principles of repose should be applied in illness when it comes in other forms than that of pain. We can easily increase whatever illness may attack us by the nervous strain which comes from fright, anxiety, or annoyance. I have seen a woman retain a severe cold for days more than was necessary, simply because of the chronic state of strain she kept herself in by fretting about it; and in another unpleasantly amusing case the sufferer's constantly expressed annoyance took the form of working almost without intermission to find remedies for herself. Without using patience enough to wait for the result of one remedy, she would rush to another until she became—so to speak—twisted and snarled in the meshes of a cold which it took weeks thoroughly to cure. This is not uncommon, and not confined merely to a cold in the head.

We can increase the suffering of friends through "sympathy" given in the same mistaken way by which we increase our own pain, or keep ourselves longer than necessary in an uncomfortable illness.

IX.

NERVOUS STRAIN IN THE EMOTIONS

THE most intense suffering which follows a misuse of the nervous power comes from exaggerated, unnecessary, or sham emotions. We each have our own emotional microscope, and the strength of its lens increases in proportion to the supersensitiveness of our nervous system. If we are a little tired, an emotion which in itself might hardly be noticed, so slight is the cause and so small the result, will be magnified many times. If we are very tired, the magnifying process goes on until often we have made ourselves ill through various sufferings, all of our own manufacture.

This increase of emotion has not always nervous fatigue as an excuse. Many people have inherited emotional magnifying glasses, and carry them through the world, getting and giving unnecessary pain, and losing more than half of the delight of life in failing to get an unprejudiced view of it. If the tired man or woman would have the good sense to stop for one minute and use the power which is given us all of understanding and appreciating our own perverted states and so move on to better, how easy it would be to recognize that a feeling is exaggerated because of fatigue, and wait until we have gained the power to drop our emotional microscopes and save all the evil results of allowing nervous excitement to control us. We are even permitted to see clearly an inherited tendency to magnify emotions and to overcome it to such an extent that life seems new to us. This must be done by the individual himself, through a personal appreciation of his own

33

mistakes and active steps to free himself from them. No amount of talking, persuading, or teaching will be of the slightest service until that personal recognition comes. This has been painfully proved too often by those who see a friend suffering unnecessarily, and in the short-sighted attempt to wrench the emotional microscope from his hand, simply cause the hold to tighten and the magnifying power to increase. A careful, steady training of the physique opens the way for a better practice of the wholesome philosophy, and the microscope drops with the relaxation of the external tension which has helped to hold it.

Emotions are often not even exaggerated but are from the beginning imaginary; and there are no more industrious imps of evil than these sham feelings. The imps have no better field for their destructive work than in various forms of morbid, personal attachment, and in what is commonly called religion,—but which has no more to do with genuine religion than the abnormal personal likings have to do with love.

It is a fact worthy of notice that the two powers most helpful, most strengthening, when sincerely felt and realized, are the ones oftenest perverted and shammed, through morbid states and abnormal nervous excitement. The sham is often so perfect an image of the reality that even the shammer is deceived.

To tell one of these pseudo-religious women that the whole attitude of her externally sanctified life is a sham emotion, would rouse anything but a saintly spirit, and surprise her beyond measure. Yet the contrast between the true, healthful, religious feeling and the sham is perfectly marked, even though both classes follow the same forms and belong to the same charitable societies. With the one, religion seems to be an accomplishment, with a rivalry as to who can carry it to the finest point; with the other, it is a steadily growing power of wholesome use.

This nervous strain from sham emotions, it must be confessed, is more common to the feminine nature. So dangerously prevalent is it that in every girls' school a true repression of the sham and a development of real feeling should be the thoughtful, silent effort of all the teachers. Any one who knows young girls feels deeply the terrible harm which comes to them in the weakening of their delicate, nervous systems through morbid, emotional excitement. The emotions are vividly real to the girls, but entirely sham in themselves. Great care must be taken to respect the sense of reality which a young girl has in these mistakes, until she can be led out so far that she herself recognizes the sham; then will come a hearty, wholesome desire to be free from it.

A school governed by a woman with strong "magnetism," and an equally strong love of admiration and devotion, can be kept in a chronic state of hysteria by the emotional affection of the girls for their teacher. When they cannot reach the teacher they will transfer the feeling to one another. Where this is allowed to pervade the atmosphere of a girls' school, those who escape floods of tears or other acute hysterical symptoms are the dull, phlegmatic temperaments.

Often a girt will go from one of these morbid attachments to another, until she seems to have lost the power for a good, wholesome affection. Strange as it may seem, the process is a steady hardening of the heart. The same result comes to man or woman who has followed a series of emotional flirtations,—the perceptions are dulled, and the whole tone of the system, mental and physical, is weakened. The effect is in exact correspondence in another degree with the result which follows an habitual use of stimulants.

Most abnormal emotional states are seen in women—and sometimes in men—who believe themselves in love. The suffering is to them very real. It seems cruel to say, "My dear, you are not in the least in love with that man; you are in love with your own emotions. If some one more attractive should appear, you could at once transfer your emotional tortures to the seemingly more worthy object." Such ideas need not be flung in so many words at a woman, but she may be gently led until she sees clearly for herself the mistake, and will even laugh at the morbid sensations that before seemed to her terribly real.

How many foolish, almost insane actions of men and women come from sham emotions and the nervous excitement generated by them, or from nervous excitement and the sham emotions that result in consequence!

Care should be taken first to change the course of the nervous power that is expressing itself morbidly, to open for it a healthy outlet, to guide it into that more wholesome channel, and then help the owner to a better control and a clearer understanding, that she may gain a healthy use of her wonderful nervous power. A gallop on horseback, a good swim, fresh air taken with any form of wholesome fun and exercise is the way to begin if possible. A woman who has had all the fresh air and interesting exercise she needs, will shake off the first sign of morbid emotions as she would shake off a rat or any other vermin.

To one who is interested to study the possible results of misdirected nervous power, nothing could illustrate it with more painful force than the story by Rudyard Kipling, "In the Matter of a Private."

Real emotions, whether painful or delightful, leave one eventually with a new supply of strength; the sham, without exception, leave their victim weaker, physically and mentally, unless they are recognized as sham, and voluntarily dismissed by the owner of the nerves that have been rasped by them. It is an inexpressibly sad sight to see a woman broken, down and an invalid, for no reason whatever but the unnecessary nervous excitement of weeks and months of sham emotion. Hardly too strong an appeal can be made to mothers and teachers for a careful watchfulness of their girls, that their emotions be kept steadily wholesome, so that they may grow and develop into that great power for use and healthful sympathy which always belongs to a woman of fine feeling.

There is a term used in college which describes most expressively an intense nervous excitement and want of control,—namely, "dry drunk." It has often seemed to me that sham emotions are a woman's form of getting drunk, and nervous prostration is its delirium tremens. Not the least of the suffering caused by emotional excitement comes from mistaken sympathy with others. Certain people seem to live on the principle that if a friend is in a swamp, it is necessary to plunge in with him; and that if the other man is up to his waist, the sympathizer shows his friendliness by allowing the mud to come up to his neck. Whereas, it is evident that the deeper my friend is immersed in a swamp, the more sure I must be to keep on firm ground that I may help him out; and sometimes I cannot even give my hand, but must use a long pole, the more surely to relieve him from danger. It is the same with a mental or moral swamp, or most of all with a nervous swamp, and yet so little do people appreciate the use of this long pole that if I do not cry when my friend cries, moan when my friend moans, and persistently refuse to plunge into the same grief that I may be of more real use in helping him out of it, I am accused by my friend and my friend's friend of coldness and want of sympathy. People have been known to refuse the other end of your pole because you will not leave it and come into the swamp with them.

It is easy to see why this mistaken sympathy is the cause of great unnecessary nervous strain. The head nurse of a hospital in one of our large cities was interrupted while at dinner by the deep interest taken by the other nurses in seeing an accident case brought in. When the man was put out of sight the nurses lost their appetite from sympathy; and the forcible way with which their superior officer informed them that if they had any real sympathy for the man they would eat to gain strength to serve him, gave a lesson by which many nervous sympathizers could greatly profit.

Of course it is possible to become so hardened that you "eat your dinner" from a want of feeling, and to be consumed only with sympathy for yourself; but it is an easy matter to make the distinction between a strong, wholesome sympathy and selfish want of feeling, and easier to distinguish between the sham sympathy and the real. The first causes you to lose nervous strength, the second gives you new power for wholesome use to others.

In all the various forms of nervous strain, which we study to avoid, let us realize and turn from false sympathy as one to be especially and entirely shunned.

Sham emotions are, of course, always misdirected force; but it is not unusual to see a woman suffering from nervous prostration caused by nervous power lying idle. This form of invalidism comes to women who have not enough to fill their lives in necessary interest and work, and have not thought of turning or been willing to turn their attention to some needed charity or work for others. A woman in this state is like a steam-engine with the fire in full blast, and the boiler shaking with the power of steam not allowed to escape in motive force.

A somewhat unusual example of this is a young woman who had been brought up as a nervous invalid, had been through nervous prostration once, and was about preparing for another attack, when she began to work for a better control of her nervous force. After gaining a better use of her machine, she at once applied its power to work,— gradually at first and then more and more, until she found herself able to endure what others had to give up as beyond their strength.

The help for these, and indeed for all cases, is to make the life objective instead of subjective. "Look out, not in;

look up, not down; lend a hand," is the motto that must be followed gently and gradually, but *surely,* to cure or to prevent a case of "Americanitis."

But again, good sense and care must be taken to preserve the equilibrium; for nervous tension and all the suffering that it brings come more often from mistaken devotion to others than from a want of care for them. Too many of us are trying to make special Providences of ourselves for our friends. To say that this short-sighted martyrdom is not only foolish but selfish seems hard, but a little thought will show it to be so.

A woman sacrifices her health in over-exertion for a friend. If she does not distress the object of her devotion entirely out of proportion to the use she performs, she at least unfits herself, by over-working, for many other uses, and causes more suffering than she saves. So are the great ends sacrificed to the smaller.

"If you only knew how hard I am trying to do right" comes with a strained face and nervous voice from many and many a woman. If she could only learn in this case, as in others, of "vaulting ambition that o'er-leaps itself and falls upon the other side;" if she could only realize that the very strained effort with which she tries, makes it impossible for her to gain,—if she would only "relax" to whatever she has to do, and then try, the gain would be incomparable.

The most intense sufferers from nervous excitement are those who suppress any sign of their feeling. The effort to "hold in" increases the nervous strain immensely. As in the case of one etherized, who has suppressed fright which he feels very keenly, as soon as the voluntary muscles are relaxed the impression on the brain shows itself with all the vehemence of the feeling,—so when the muscles are consciously relaxed the nervous excitement bursts forth like the eruption of a small volcano, and for a time is a surprise to the man or woman who has been in a constant effort of suppression.

The contrast between true self-control and that which is merely repressed feeling, is, like all contrast between the natural and the artificial, immeasurable; and the steadily increasing power to be gained by true self-control cannot be conveyed in words, but must be experienced in actual use.

Many of us know with what intense force a temper masters us when, having held in for some time, some spring is touched which makes silence impossible, and the sense of relief which follows a volley of indignant words. To say that we can get a far greater and more lasting relief without a word, but simply through relaxing our muscles and freeing our excited nerves, seems tame; but it is practically true, and is indeed the only way from a physical standpoint that one may be sure of controlling a high temper. In that way, also, we keep the spirit, the power, the strength, from which the temper comes, and so far from being tame, life has more for us. We do not tire ourselves and lose nervous force through the wear and tear of losing our temper. To speak expressively, if not scientifically, Let go, and let the temper slip over your nerves and off,—you do not lose it then, for you know where it is, and you keep all the nervous force that would have been used in suppression or expression for better work.

That, the reader will say, is not so easy as it sounds. Granted, there must be the desire to get a true control of the temper; but most of us have that desire, and while we cannot expect immediate success, steady practice will bring startling results sooner than we realize. There must be a clear, intelligent understanding of what we are aiming at, and how to gain it; but that is not difficult, and once recognized grows steadily as we gain practical results. Let the first feeling of anger be a reminder to "let go." But you will say, "I do not want to let go,"—only because your various grandfathers and grandmothers were unaccustomed to relieving themselves in that manner. When we give way to anger and let it out in a volley of words, there is often a sense of relief, but more often a reaction which is most unpleasant, and is greatly increased by the pain given to others. The relief is certain if we "relax;" and not only is there then no painful reaction, but we gain a clear head to recognize the justice or injustice of our indignation, and to see what can be done about its cause.

Petty irritability can be met in the same way. As with nervous pain it seems at first impossible to "relax to it;" but the Rubicon once crossed, we cannot long be irritable,—it is so much simpler not to be, and so much more comfortable.

If when we are tempted to fly into a rage or to snap irritably at others we could go through a short process of relaxing motions, the effect would be delightful. But that would be ridiculous; and we must do our relaxing in the privacy of the closet and recall it when needed outside, that we may relax without observation except in its happy results. I know people will say that anything to divert the mind will cure a high temper or irritability. That is only so to a limited extent; and so far as it is so, simply proves the best process of control. Diversion relieves the nervous excitement, turning the attention in another direction,—and so is relaxing so far as it goes.

Much quicker and easier than self-control is the control which allows us to meet the irritability of others without echoing it. The temptation to echo a bad temper or an irritable disposition in others, we all know; but the relief which comes to ourselves and to the sufferer as we quietly relax and refuse to reflect it, is a sensation that many of us have yet to experience. One keeps a clear head in that way, not to mention a charitable heart; saves any quantity of nervous strain, and keeps off just so much tendency to nervous prostration.

Practically the way is opened to this better control through a physical training which gives us the power of relaxing at will, and so of maintaining a natural, wholesome equilibrium of nerves and muscles.

Personal sensitiveness is, to a great degree, a form of nervous tension. An individual case of the relief of this sensitiveness, although laughable in the means of cure, is so perfectly illustrative of it that it is worth telling. A lady who suffered very much from having her feelings hurt came to me for advice. I told her whenever anything was said to wound her, at once to imagine her legs heavy,—that relaxed her muscles, freed her nerves, and relieved the tension caused by her sensitive feelings. The cure seemed to her wonderful. It would not have done for her to think a table heavy, or a chair, or to have diverted her mind in any other way, for it was the effect of relaxation in her own body that she wanted, which came from persistently thinking her legs heavy. Neither could her sensitiveness have taken a very deep hold, or mere outside relaxation would not have reached it; but that outside process had the effect of greatly assisting in the power to use a higher philosophy with the mind.

Self-consciousness and all the personal annoyances that come with or follow it are to so great an extent nervous tension, that the ease with which they may be helped seems sometimes like a miracle to those who study for a better guidance of their bodies.

Of worries, from the big worries with a real foundation to the miserable, petty, nagging worries that wear a woman's nervous system more than any amount of steady work, there is so much to be said that it would prove tedious, and indeed unnecessary to recount them. A few words will suggest enough toward their remedy to those who are looking in the right direction, and to others many words would be of no avail.

The petty worries are the most wearing, and they fortunately are the most easily helped. By relaxing the muscular contractions invariably accompanying them we seem to make an open channel, and they slip through,— which expression I am well aware is not scientific. The common saying, "Cares roll off her like water off a duck's back," means the same thing. Some human ducks are made with backs eminently fitted for cares to slip from; but those whose backs seem to be made to hold the cares can remould themselves to the right proportions, and there is great compensation in their appreciation of the contrast.

Never resist a worry. It is increased many times by the effort to overcome it. The strain of the effort makes it constantly more difficult to drop the strain of the worry. When we quietly go to work to relax the muscles and so quiet the nerves, ignoring a worry, the way in which it disappears is surprising. Then is the time to meet it with a broad philosophizing on the uselessness of worry, etc., and "clinch" our freedom, so to speak.

It is not at the first attempt to relax, or the second, or the ninth, that the worry will disappear for many of us, and especially for worriers. It takes many hours to learn what relaxing is; but having once learned, its helpful power is too evident for us not to keep at it, if we really desire to gain our freedom.

To give the same direction to a worrier that was so effective with the woman whose feelings were easily hurt, may seem equally ridiculous; but in many cases it will certainly prove most useful. When you begin to worry, think your legs heavy. Your friends will appreciate the relief more than you do, and will gain as you gain.

A recital of all the emotional disturbances which seem to have so strong a hold on us, and which are merely misdirected nervous force, might easily fill a volume; but a few of the most common troubles, such as have been given, will perhaps suffice to help each individual to understand his own especial temptations in that direction,—and if I have made even partially clear the ease with which they may be relieved through careful physical training, it is all I can hope for.

The body must be trained to obey the mind; the mind must be trained to give the body commands worth obeying.

The real feelings of life are too exquisite and strengthening in their depth and power to be crowded out by those gross forms of nervous excitement which I can find no better name for than sham emotions. If we could only realize this more broadly, and bring up the children with a wholesome dread of morbid feeling what a marked change would there be in the state of the entire race!

All physicians agree that in most cases it is not overwork, it is not mental strain, that causes the greater number of cases of nervous disturbance, but that they are more often brought on by emotional strain.

The deepest grief, as well as the greatest joy, can be met in a way to give new strength and new power for use if we have a sound philosophy and a well-guided, wholesome body to meet it. But these last are the work of years; and neither the philosophy nor the physical strength can be brought to bear at short notice, although we can do much toward a better equilibrium even late in life.

Various forms of egotism, if not exactly sham emotions, are the causes of great nervous strain. Every physician knows the intense egotism which often comes with nervous prostration. Some one has very aptly said that insanity is only egotism gone to seed. It often seems so, especially when it begins with nervous prostration. We cannot be too careful to shun this nervous over-care for self.

We inherit so strongly the subjective way of living rather than the objective, that it impresses itself upon our very nerves; and they, instead of being open channels for the power always at our command to pass freely to the use for which it is intended, stop the way by means of the attention which is so uselessly turned back on ourselves, our narrow personal interests, and our own welfare. How often we see cases where by means of the nervous tension all this has increased to a disease, and the tiresome *Ego* is a monster in the way of its owner and all his would-be friends. "I cannot bear this." "I shall take cold." "If you only knew how I suffered." Why should we know, unless through knowing we can give you some relief? And so it goes, I—I—I— forever, and the more the more nervous prostration.

Keep still, that all which is good may come to you, and live out to others that your life may broaden for use. In this way we can take all that Nature is ready to give us, and will constantly give us, and use it as hers and for her purposes, which are always the truest and best Then we live as a little child would live,—only with more wisdom.

X.

NATURE'S TEACHING

NATURE is not only our one guide in the matter of physical training, she is the chief engineer who will keep us in order and control the machine, if we aim to fulfil her conditions and shun every personal interference with the wholesome working of her laws.

Here is where the exquisite sense of growing power comes. In studying Nature, we not only realize the strength that comes from following her lead, but we discover her in ourselves gently moving us onward.

We all believe we look to Nature, if we think at all; and it is a surprise to find how mistaken we are. The time would not be wasted if we whose duties do not lead us to any direct study of natural life for personal reasons, would take fifteen minutes every day simply to think of Nature and her methods of working, and to see at the same time where, so far as we individually are concerned, we constantly interfere with the best use of her powers. With all reverence I say it, this should be the first form of prayer; and our ability to pray sincerely to God and live in accordance with His laws would grow in proportion to our power of sincere sympathy with the workings of those laws in Nature.

Try to realize the quiet power of all natural growth and movement, from a blade of grass, through a tree, a forest of trees, the entire vegetable growth on the earth, the movement of the planets, to the growth and involuntary vital operations of our own bodies.

No words can bring so full a realization of the quiet power in the progress of Nature as will the simple process of following the growth of a tree in imagination from the working of its sap in the root up to the tips of the leaves, the blossoms, and the fruit. Or beginning lower, follow the growth of a blade of grass or a flower, then a tree, and so on to the movement of the earth, and then of all the planets in the universe. Let your imagination picture so vividly all natural movements, little by little, that you seem to be really at one with each and all. Study the orderly working of your own bodily functions; and having this clearly in mind, notice where you, in all movements that are or might be under the control of your will, are disobeying Nature's laws.

Nature shows us constantly that at the back of every action there should be a great repose. This holds good from the minutest growth to the most powerful tornado. It should be so with us not only in the simple daily duties, but in all things up to the most intense activity possible to man. And this study and realization of Nature's method which I am pleading for brings a vivid sense of our own want of repose. The compensation is fortunately great, or the discouragement might be more than could be borne. We must appreciate a need to have it supplied; we must see a mistake in order to shun it.

How can we expect repose of mind when we have not even repose of muscle? When the most external of the machine is not at our command, surely the spirit that animates the whole cannot find its highest plane of action. Or how can we possibly expect to know the repose that should be at our command for every emergency, or hope to realize the great repose behind every action, when we have not even learned the repose in rest?

Think of Nature's resting times, and see how painful would be the result of a digression.

Our side of the earth never turns suddenly toward the sun at night, giving us flashes of day in the darkness. When it is night, it is night steadily, quietly, until the time comes for day. A tree in winter, its time for rest, never starts out with a little bud here and there, only to be frost bitten, and so when spring-time comes, to result in an uneven looking, imperfectly developed tree. It rests entirely in its time for rest; and when its time for blooming comes, its action is full and true and perfect. The grass never pushes itself up in little, untimely blades through the winter, thus leaving our lawns and fields full of bare patches in the warmer season. The flowers that close at night do not half close, folding some petals and letting others stay wide open. Indeed, so perfectly does Nature rest when it is her time for resting, that even the suggestion of these abnormal actions seems absolutely ridiculous. The less we allow ourselves to be controlled by Nature's laws, the more we ignore their wonderful beauty; and yet there is that in us which must constantly respond to Nature unconsciously, else how could we at once feel the absurdity of any disobedience to her laws, everywhere except with man? And man, who is not only free to obey, but has exquisite and increasing power to realize and enjoy them in all their fulness, lives so far out of harmony with these laws as ever to be blind to his own steady disobedience.

Think of the perfect power for rest in all animals. Lift a cat when she is quiet, and see how perfectly relaxed she is in every muscle. That is not only the way she sleeps, but the way she rests; and no matter how great or how rapid the activity, she drops all tension at once when she stops. So it is with all animals, except in rare cases where man has tampered with them in a way to interfere with the true order of their lives.

Watch a healthy baby sleeping; lift its arm, its leg, or its head carefully, and you will find each perfectly relaxed and free. You can even hold it on your outspread hands, and the whole little weight, full of life and gaining new power through the perfect rest, will give itself entirely to your hands, without one particle of tension. The sleep that we get in babyhood is the saving health of many. But, alas! at a very early age useless tension begins, and goes on increasing; and if it does not steadily lead to acute "Americanitis," it prevents the perfect use of all our powers. Mothers, watch your children with a care which will be all the more effective because they will be unconscious of it; for a child's attention should seldom be drawn to its own body. Lead them toward the laws of Nature, that they may grow in harmony with them, and so be saved the useless suffering, strain, and trouble that comes to us Americans. If we do not take care, the children will more and more inherit this fearful misuse of the nervous force, and the inheritance will be so strong that at best we can have only little invalids. How great the necessity seems for the effort to get back into Nature's ways when we reflect upon the possibilities of a continued disobedience!

To be sure, Nature has Repose itself and does not have to work for it. Man is left free to take it or not as he chooses. But before he is able to receive it he has personal tendencies to restlessness to overcome. And more than that, there are the inherited nervous habits of generations of ancestors to be recognized and shunned. But repose is an inmost law of our being, and the quiet of Nature is at our command much sooner than we realize, if we want it enough to work for it steadily day by day. Nothing will increase our realization of the need more than a little daily thought of the quiet in the workings of Nature and the consequent appreciation of our own lack. Ruskin tells the story with his own expressive power when he says, "Are not the elements of ease on the face of all the greatest works of creation? Do they not say, not there has been a great *effort* here, but there has been a great power here?"

The greatest act, the only action which we know to be power in itself, is the act of Creation. Behind that action there lies a great Repose. We are part of Creation, we should be moved by its laws. Let us shun everything we see to be in the way of our own best power of action in muscle, nerve, senses, mind, and heart. Who knows the new perception and strength, the increased power for use that is open to us if we will but cease to be an obstruction?

Freedom within the limits of Nature's laws, and indeed there is no freedom without those limits, is best studied and realized in the growth of all plants,—in the openness of the branch of a vine to receive the sap from the main stem, in the free circulation of the sap in a tree and in all vegetable organisms.

Imagine the branch of a vine endowed with the power to grow according to the laws which govern it, or to ignore and disobey those laws. Imagine the same branch having made up its vegetable mind that it could live its own life apart from the vine, twisting its various fibres into all kinds of knots and snarls, according to its own idea of living, so that the sap from the main stem could only reach it in a minimum quantity. What a dearth of leaf, flower, and fruit would appear in the branch! Yet the figure is perfectly illustrative of the way in which most of us are interfering with the best use of the life that is ours.

Freedom is obedience to law. A bridge can be built to stand, only in obedience to the laws of mechanics. Electricity can be made a useful power only in exact obedience to the laws that govern it, otherwise it is most destructive. Has man the privilege of disobeying natural laws, only in the use of his own individual powers? Clearly not. And why is it that while recognizing and endeavoring to obey the laws of physics, of mechanics, and all other laws of Nature in his work in the world, he so generally defies the same laws in their application to his own being?

The freedom of an animal's body in obeying the animal instincts is beautiful to watch. The grace and power expressed in the freedom of a tiger are wonderful. The freedom in the body of a baby to respond to every motion and expression is exquisite to study. But before most children have been in the world three years their inherited personal contractions begin, and unless the little bodies can be watched and trained out of each unnecessary contraction as it appears, and so kept in their own freedom, there comes a time later, when to live to the greatest power for use they must spend hours in learning to be babies all over again, and then gain a new freedom and natural movement.

The law which perhaps appeals to us most strongly when trying to identify ourselves with Nature is the law of rhythm: action, re-action; action, re-action; action, re-action,—and the two must balance, so that equilibrium is always the result. There is no similar thought that can give us keener pleasure than when we rouse all our imagination, and realize all our power of identifying ourselves with the workings of a great law, and follow this rhythmic movement till we find rhythm within rhythm,—from the rhythmic motion of the planets to the delicate vibrations of heat and light. It is helpful to think of rhythmic growth and motion, and not to allow the thought of a new rhythm to pass without identifying ourselves with it as fully as our imagination will allow.

We have the rhythm of the seasons, of day and night, of the tides, and of vegetable and animal life,—as the various rhythmic motions in the flying of birds. The list will be endless, of course, for the great law rules everything in Nature, and our appreciation of it grows as we identify ourselves with its various modes of action.

One hair's variation in the rhythm of the universe would bring destruction, and yet we little individual microcosms are knocking ourselves into chronic states of chaos because we feel that we can be gods, and direct our own lives so much better than the God who made us. We are left in freedom to go according to His laws, or against them; and we are generally so convinced that our own stupid, short-sighted way is the best, that it is only because Nature tenderly holds to some parts of us and keeps them in the rhythm, that we do not hurl ourselves to pieces. *This law of rhythm—or of equilibrium in motion and in rest—is the end, aim, and effect of all true physical training for the development and guidance of the body.* Its ruling power is proved in the very construction of the body,—the two sides; the circulation of the blood, veins and arteries; the muscles, extensor and flexor; the nerves, sensory and motor.

When the long rest of a body balances the long activity, in day and night; when the shorter rests balance the shorter activity, as in the various opportunities offered through the day for entire rest, if only a minute at a time; when the sensory and motor nerves are clear for impression and expression; when the muscles in parts of the body not needed are entirely quiet, allowing those needed for a certain action to do their perfect work; when the co-ordination of the muscles in use is so established that the force for a movement is evenly divided; when the flexor rests while its antagonizing muscle works, and *vice versa,*—when all this which is merely a *natural power for action and rest* is automatically established, then the body is ready to obey and will obey the lightest touch of its owner, going in whatever direction it may be sent, artistic, scientific, or domestic. As this exquisite sense of ease in a natural movement grows upon us, no one can describe the feeling of new power or of positive comfort which comes with it; and yet it is no miracle, it is only natural. The beasts have the same freedom; but they have not the mind to put it to higher uses, or the sense to enjoy its exquisite power.

Often it seems that the care and trouble to get back into Nature's way is more than compensated for in the new appreciation of her laws and their uses. But the body, after all, is merely a servant; and, however perfect its training may have been, if the man, the master, puts his natural power to mean or low uses, sooner or later the power will be lost. Self-conscious pride will establish its own contractions. The use of a natural power for evil ends will limit itself sooner or later. The love for unwholesome surroundings will eventually put a check on a perfectly free body, although sometimes the wonder is that the check is so long in coming. If we have once trained ourselves into natural ways, so akin are the laws of Nature and spirit, both must be obeyed; and to rise to our greatest power means always to rise to our greatest power for use. "A man's life is God's love for the use for which he was made;" a man's power lies in the best direction of that use. This is a truth as practical as the necessity for walking on the feet with the head up.

XI.

THE CHILD AS AN IDEAL

WHILE the path of progress in the gaining of repose could not be traced thus far without reference to the freedom of a baby, a fuller consideration of what we may learn from this source must be of great use to us.

The peace and freshness of a little baby are truly beautiful, but are rarely appreciated. Few of us have peace enough in ourselves to respond to these charms. It is like playing the softest melody upon a harp to those whose ears have long been closed.

Let us halt, and watch, and listen, and see what we shall gain!

Throughout the muscular system of a normal, new-born baby it is impossible to find any waste of force. An apparent waste will, upon examination, prove itself otherwise. Its cry will at first seem to cause contractions of the face; but the absolute removal of all traces of contraction as the cry ceases, and a careful watching of the act itself, show it to be merely an exaggeration of muscular action, not a permanent contraction. Each muscle is balanced by an opposing one; in fact, the whole thing is only a very even stretching of the face, and, undoubtedly, has a purpose to accomplish.

Examine a baby's bed, and see how distinctly it bears the impression of an absolute giving up of weight and power. They actually *do* that which we only theorize about, and from them we may learn it all, if we will.

A babe in its bath gives us another fine opportunity for learning to be simple and free. It yields to the soft pressure of the water with a repose which is deeply expressive of gratitude; while we, in our clumsy departures from Nature's state, often resist with such intensity as not to know—in circumstances just as simply useful to us—that we have anything for which to be grateful.

In each new experience we find it the same, the healthy baby yields, *lets himself go,* with an case which must double his chances for comfort. Could we but learn to do so, our lives would lengthen, and our joys and usefulness strengthen in exact proportion.

All through the age of unconsciousness, this physical freedom is maintained even where the mental attitude is not free. Baby wrath is as free and economical of physical force as are the winsome moods, and this until the personality has developed to some extent,—that is, *until the child reflects the contractions of those around him.* It expends itself in well-balanced muscular exercise, one set of muscles resting fully in their moment of non-use, while another set takes up the battle. At times it will seem that all wage war together; if so, the rest is equal to the action.

It is not the purpose of this chapter to recommend anger, even of the most approved sort; but if we will express the emotion at all, let us do it as well as we did in our infancy!

Channels so free as this would necessitate, would lessen our temptations to such expression; we, with mature intellects, would see it for what it is, and the next generation of babies would less often exercise their wonderfully balanced little bodies in such an unlovely waste.

Note the perfect openness of a baby throat as the child coos out his expression of happiness. Could anything be more free, more like the song of a bird in its obedience to natural laws? Alas, for how much must we answer that these throats are so soon contracted, the tones changed to so high

58

a pitch, the voice becoming so shrill and harsh! Can we not open our throats and become as these little children?

The same *openness* in the infant organism is the child's protection in many dangers. Falls that would result in breaks, strains, or sprains in us, leave the baby entirely whole save in its "feelings," and often there, too, if the child has been kept in the true state mentally.

Watch a baby take its food, and contrast it with our own ways of eating. The baby draws it in slowly and evenly, with a quiet rhythm which is in exact accord with the rhythmic action of its digestive organs. You feel each swallow taken in the best way for repair, and for this reason it seems sometimes as if one could see a baby grow while feeding. There cannot be a lovelier glimpse of innocent physical repose than the little respites from the fatigue of feeding which a baby often takes. His face moist, with open pores, serene and satisfied, he views the hurry about him as an interesting phase of harmless madness. He is entirely outside of it until self-consciousness is quite developed.

The sleep of a little child is another opportunity for us to learn what we need. Every muscle free, every burden dropped, each breath carries away the waste, and fills its place with the needed substance of increasing growth and power.

In play, we find the same freedom. When one idea is being executed, every other is excluded. They do not think *dolls* while they roll *hoop!*

They do not think of work while they play. Examine and see how we do both. The baby of one year, sitting on the shore burying his fat hand in the soft warm sand, is for the time being alive *only* to its warmth and softness, with a dim consciousness of the air and color about him. If we could engross ourselves as fully and with as simple a pleasure, we should know far more of the possible power of our minds for both work and rest.

It is interesting to watch normal children in these concentrations, because from their habits we may learn so much which may improve our own sadly different manner of living. It is also interesting but pathetic to see the child gradually leaving them as he approaches boyhood, and to trace our part in leading him away from the true path.

The baby's perfect placidity, caused by mental and bodily freedom, is disturbed at a very early age by those who should be his true guides. It would be impossible to say when the first wrong impression is made, but it is so early that a true statement of the time could only be accepted from scientific men. For mothers and fathers have often so dulled their own sensitiveness, that they are powerless to recognize the needs of their children, and their impressions are, in consequence, untrustworthy.

At the time the pangs of teething begin, it is the same. The healthy child left to itself would wince occasionally at the slight pricking pain, and then turn its entire attention elsewhere, and thus become refreshed for the next trial. But under the adult influence the agony of the first little prick is often magnified until the result is a cross, tired baby, already removed several degrees from the beautiful state of peace and freedom in which Nature placed him under our care.

The bodily freedom of little children is the foundation of a most beautiful mental freedom, which cannot be wholly destroyed by us. This is plainly shown by the childlike trust which they display in all the affairs of life, and also in their exquisite responsiveness to the spiritual truths which are taught to them. The very expression of face of a little child as it is led by the hand is a lesson to us upon which pages might be written.

Had we the same spirit dwelling in us, we more often should feel ourselves led "beside the still waters," and made "to lie down in green pastures." We should grow faster spiritually, because we should not make conflicts for ourselves, but should meet with the Lord's quiet strength whatever we had to pass through.

Let us learn of these little ones, and help them to hold fast to that which they teach us. Let us remember that the natural and the ideal are truly one, and endeavor to reach the latter by means of the former.

When through hereditary tendency our little child is not ideal,—that is, natural,—let us with all the more earnestness learn to be quiet ourselves that we may lead him to it, and thus open the channels of health and strength.

XII.

TRAINING FOR REST

BUT how shall we gain a natural repose? It is absurd to emphasize the need without giving the remedy. "I should be so glad to relax, but I do not know how," is the sincere lament of many a nervously strained being.

There is a regular training which acts upon the nervous force and teaches its proper use, as the gymnasium develops the muscles. This, as will be easily seen, is at first just the reverse of vigorous exercise, and no woman should do powerful muscular work without learning at the same time to guide her body with true economy of force. It is appalling to watch the faces of women in a gymnasium, to see them using five, ten, twenty times the nervous force necessary for every exercise. The more excited they get, the more nervous force they use; and the hollows under their eyes increase, the strained expression comes, and then they wonder that after such fascinating exercise they feel so tired. A common sight in gymnasium work, especially among women, is the nervous straining of the muscles of the arms and hands, while exercises meant for the legs alone are taken. This same muscular tension is evident in the arm that should be at rest while the other arm is acting; and if this want of equilibrium in exercise is so strikingly noticeable in the limbs themselves, how much worse it must be all through the less prominent muscles! To guide the body in trapeze work, every well-trained acrobat knows he must have a quiet mind, a clear head, and obedient muscles. I recall a woman who stands high in gymnastic work, whose agility on the triple bars is excellent, but the nervous strain shown in the drawn lines of her face before she begins, leaves one who studies her carefully always in doubt as to whether she will not get confused before her difficult performance is over, and break her neck in consequence. A realization also of the unnecessary nervous force she is using, detracts greatly from the pleasure in watching her performance.

If we were more generally sensitive to misdirected nervous power, this interesting gymnast, with many others, would lose no time in learning a more quiet and naturally economical guidance of her muscles, and gymnasium work would not be, as Dr. Checkley very justly calls it, "more often a straining than a training."

To aim a gun and hit the mark, a quiet control of the muscles is necessary. If the purpose of our actions were as well defined as the bull's eye of a target, what wonderful power in the use of our muscles we might very soon obtain! But the precision and ease in an average motion comes so far short of its possibility, that if the same carelessness were taken as a matter of course in shooting practice, the side of a barn should be an average target.

Gymnasium work for women would be grand in its wholesome influence, if only they might learn the proper *use* of the body while they are working for its development. And no gymnasium will be complete and satisfactory in its results until the leader arranges separate classes for training in economy of force and rhythmic motion. In order to establish a true physical balance the training of the nerves should receive as much attention as the training of the muscles. The more we misuse our nervous force, the worse the expenditure will be as muscular power increases; I cannot waste so much force on a poorly developed muscle as on one that is well developed. This does not by any means argue against the development of muscle; it argues for its proper use. Where is the good of an exquisitely formed machine, if it is to be shattered for want of control of the motive power?

It would of course be equally harmful to train the guiding power while neglecting entirely flabby, undeveloped muscles. The only difference is that in the motions for this training and for the perfect co-ordinate use of the muscles, there must be a certain amount of even, muscular development; whereas although the vigorous exercise for the growth of the muscles often helps toward a healthy nervous system, it more often, where the nervous force is misused, exaggerates greatly the tension.

In every case it is equilibrium we are working for, and a one-sided view of physical training is to be deplored and avoided, whether the balance is lost on the side of the nerves or the muscles.

Take a little child early enough, and watch it carefully through a course of natural rhythmic exercises, and there will be no need for the careful training necessary to older people. But help for us who have gone too far in this tension comes only through patient study.

So far as I can, I will give directions for gaining the true relaxation. But because written directions are apt to be misunderstood, and so bring discouragement and failure, I will purposely omit all but the most simple means of help;

but these I am sure will bring very pleasant effects if followed exactly and with the utmost patience.

The first care should be to realize how far you are from the ability to let go of your muscles when they are not needed; how far you are from the natural state of a cat when she is quiet, or better still from the perfect freedom of a sleeping baby; consequently how impossible it is for you ever to rest thoroughly. Almost all of us are constantly exerting ourselves to hold our own heads on. This is easily proved by our inability to let go of them. The muscles are so well balanced that Nature holds our heads on much more perfectly than we by any possibility can. So it is with all our muscles; and to teach them better habits we must lie flat on our backs, and try to give our whole weight to the floor or the bed. The floor is better, for that does not yield in the least to us, and the bed does. Once on the floor, give way to it as far as possible. Every day you will become more sensitive to tension, and every day you will be better able to drop it. While you are flat on your backs, if you can find some one to "prove" your relaxation, so much the better. Let your friend lift an arm, bending it at the different joints, and then carefully lay it down. See if you can give its weight entirely to the other person, so that it seems to be no part of you, but as separate as if it were three bags of sand, fastened loosely at the wrist, the elbow, and the shoulder; it will then be full of life without tension. You will find probably, either that you try to assist in raising the arm in your anxiety to make it heavy, or you will resist so that it is not heavy with its own weight but with I your personal effort. In some cases the nervous force is so active that the arm reminds one of a lively eel.

Then have your legs treated in the same way. It is good even to have some one throw your arm or your leg up and catch it; also to let it go unexpectedly. Unnecessary tension is proved when the limb, instead of dropping by the pure force of gravity, sticks fast wherever it was left. The remark when the extended limb is brought to the attention of its owner is, "Well, what did you want me to do? You did not say you wanted me to drop it,"—which shows the habitual attitude of tension so vividly as to be almost ridiculous; the very idea being, of course, that you are not wanted to do anything but *let go,* when the arm would drop of its own accord. If the person holding your arm says, "Now I will let go, and it must drop as if a dead weight," almost invariably it will not be the force of gravity that takes it, but your own effort to make it a dead weight; and it will come down with a thump which shows evident muscular effort, or so slowly and actively as to prove that you cannot let it alone. Constant and repeated trial, with right thought from the pupil, will be certain to bring good results, so that at least he or she can be sure of better power for rest in the limbs. Unfortunately this first gain will not last. Unless the work goes on, the legs and arms will soon be "all tightened up" again, and it will seem harder to let go than ever.

The next care must be with the head. That cannot be treated as roughly as the limbs. It can be tossed, if the tosser will surely catch it on his open hand. Never let it drop with its full weight on the floor, for the jar of the fall, if you are perfectly relaxed, is unpleasant; if you are tense, it is dangerous. At first move it slowly up and down. As with the arms, there will be either resistance or attempted assistance. It seems at times as though it were and always would be impossible to let go of your own head. Of course, if you cannot give up and let go for a friend to move it quietly up and down, you cannot let go and give way entirely to the restful power of sleep. The head must be moved up and down, from side to side, and round and round in opposite ways, gently and until its owner can let go so completely that it seems like a big ball in the hands that move it. Of course care must be taken to move it gently and never to extremes, and it will not do to trust an unintelligent person to "prove" a body in any way. Ladies' maids have been taught to do it very well, but they had in all cases to be carefully watched at first.

The example of a woman who had for years been an invalid is exceedingly interesting as showing how persistently people "hold on." Although the greater part of her time had been spent in a reclining attitude, she had not learned the very rudiments of relaxation, and could not let go of her own muscles any more easily than others who have always been in active life. Think of holding yourself on to the bed for ten years! Her maid learned to move her in the way that has been described, and after repeated practice, by the time she had reached the last movement the patient would often be sleeping like a baby. It did not cure her, of course; that was not expected. But it taught her to "relax" to a pain instead of bracing up and fighting it, and to live in a natural way so far as an organic disease and sixty years of misused and over-used force would allow.

Having relaxed the legs and arms and head, next the spine and all the muscles of the chest must be helped to relax. This is more difficult, and requires not only care but greater muscular strength in the lifter. If the one who is lifting will only remember to press hard on the floor with the feet, and put all the effort of lifting in the legs, the strain will be greatly lessened.

Take hold of the hands and lift the patient or pupil to a sitting attitude. Here, of course, if the muscles that hold the head are perfectly relaxed, the head will drop back from its own weight. Then, in letting the body back again, of course, keep hold of the hands,—*never* let go; and after it is down, if the neck has remained relaxed, the head will be back in a most uncomfortable attitude, and must be lifted and placed in the right position. It is some time before relaxation is so complete as that. At first the head and spine will come up like a ramrod, perfectly rigid and stiff. There will be the same effort either to assist or resist; the same disinclination to give up; often the same remark, "If you will tell me what you want me to do, I will do it;" the same inability to realize that the remark, and the feeling that prompts it, are entirely opposed to the principle that you are *wanted to do nothing, and to do nothing with an effort is impossible.* In lowering the body it must "give" like a bag of bones fastened loosely together and well padded. Sometimes when it is nearly down, one arm can be dropped, and the body let down the rest of the way by the other. Then it is simply giving way completely to the laws of gravity, it will fall over on the side that is not held, and only roll on its back as the other arm is dropped. Care must always be taken to arrange the head comfortably after the body is resting on the ground. Sometimes great help is given toward relaxing the muscles of the chest and spine by pushing the body up as if to roll it over, first one side and then the other, and letting it roll back from its own weight. It is always good, after helping the separate parts to a restful state, to take the body as a whole and roll it over and over, carefully, and see if the owner can let you do so without the slightest effort to assist you. It will be easily seen that the power, once gained, of remaining perfectly passive while another moves you, means a steadily increasing ability to relax at all times when the body should be given to perfect rest. This power to "let go" causes an increasing sensitiveness to all tension, which, unpleasant as it always is to find mistakes of any kind in ourselves, brings a very happy result in the end; for we can never shun evils, physical or spiritual, until we have recognized them fully, and every mistaken way of using our machine, when studiously avoided, brings us nearer to that beautiful unconscious use of it which makes it possible for us to forget it entirely in giving it the more truly to its highest use.

After having been helped in some degree by another, and often without that preliminary help, come the motions by which we are enabled to free ourselves; and it is interesting to see how much more easily the body will move after following this course of exercises. Take the same attitude on the floor, giving up entirely in every part to the force of gravity, and keep your eyes closed through the whole process. Then stop and imagine yourself heavy. First think one leg heavy, then the other, then each arm, and both arms, being sure to keep the same weight in the legs; then your body and head. Use your imagination to the full extent of its power, and think the whole machine heavy; wonder how the floor can hold such a weight. Begin then to take a deep breath. Inhale through the nose quietly and easily. Let it seem as if the lungs expanded themselves with, out voluntary effort on your part. Fill first the lower lungs and then the upper. Let go, and exhale the air with a sense of relief. As the air leaves your lungs, try to let your body rest back on the floor more heavily, as a rubber bag would if the air were allowed to escape from it. Repeat this breathing exercise several times; then inhale and exhale rhythmically, with breaths long enough to give about six to a minute, for ten times, increasing the number every day until you reach fifty. This eventually will establish the habit of longer breaths in the regular unconscious movement of our lungs, which is most helpful to a wholesome physical state. The directions for deep breathing should be carefully followed in the deep breaths taken after each motion. After the deep breathing, drag your leg up slowly, very slowly, trying to have no effort except in the hip joint, allowing the knee to bend, and dragging the heel heavily along the floor, until it is up so far that the sole of the foot touches without effort on your part. Stop occasionally in the motion and let the weight come into the heel, then drag the foot with less effort than before,—so will the strain of movement be steadily decreased. Let the leg slip slowly down, and when it is nearly flat on the floor again, let go, so that it gives entirely and drops from its own weight. If it is perfectly free, there is a pleasant little spring from the impetus of dropping, which is more or less according to the healthful state of the body. The same motion must be repeated with the other leg. Every movement should be slower each day. It is well to repeat the movements of the legs for three times, trying each time to move more slowly, with the leg heavier than the time before. After this, lift the arm slowly from the shoulder, letting the hand hang over until it is perpendicular to the floor. Be careful to think the arm heavy, and the motive power in the shoulder. It helps to relax if you imagine your arm held to the shoulder by a single hair, and that if you move it with a force beyond the minimum needed to raise it, it will drop off entirely. To those who have little or no imagination this will seem ridiculous; to others who have more, and can direct it usefully, this and similar ways will be very helpful. After the arm is raised to a perpendicular position, let the force of gravity have it,—first the upper arm to the elbow, and then the forearm and hand, so that it falls by pieces. Follow the same motion with the other arm, and repeat this three times, trying to improve with each repetition.

Next, the head must be moved slowly,—so slowly that it seems as though it hardly moved at all,—first rolled to the left, then back and to the right and back again; and this also can be repeated three times. After each of the above motions there should be two or three long, quiet breaths. To free the spine, sit up on the floor, and with heavy arms and legs, head dropped forward, let it go back slowly and easily, as if the vertebrae were beads on a string, and first one bead lay flat, then another and another, until the whole string rests on the floor, and the head falls back with its own weight. This should be practised over and over before the movement can be perfectly free; and it is well to begin on the bed, until you catch the idea and its true application. After, and sometimes before, the process of slow motions, rolling over loosely on one side should be practised,—remaining there until the weight all seems near the floor, and then giving way so that the force of gravity seems to "flop" it back (I use "flop" advisedly); so again resting on the other side. But one must go over by regular motions, raising the leg first heavily and

71

letting it fall with its full weight over the other leg, so that the ankles are crossed. The arm on the same side must be raised as high as possible and dropped over the chest. Then the body can be rolled over, and carried as it were by the weight of the arm and leg. It must go over heavily and freely like a bag of loose bones, and it helps greatly to freedom to roll over and over in this way.

Long breaths, taken deeply and quietly, should be interspersed all through these exercises for extreme relaxation. They prevent the possibility of relaxing too far. And as there is a pressure on every muscle of the body during a deep inspiration, the muscles, being now relaxed into freedom, are held in place, so to speak, by the pressure from the breath,—as we blow in the fingers of a glove to put them in shape.

Remember always that it is equilibrium we are working for, and this extreme relaxation will bring it, because we have erred so far in the opposite direction. For instance, there is now no balance at all between our action and our rest, because we are more or less tense and consequently active all through the times when we should be entirely at rest; and we never can be moved by Nature's rhythm until we learn absolute relaxation for rest, and so gain the true equilibrium in that way. Then again, since we use so much unnecessary tension in everything we do, although we cannot remove it entirely until we learn the normal motion of our muscles, still after an hour's practice and the consequent gain in extreme relaxation, it will be impossible to attack our work with the same amount of unnecessary force, at least for a time; and every day the time in which we are able to work, or talk, or move with less tension will increase, and so our bad habits be gradually changed, if not to good, to better ones. So the true equilibrium comes gradually more and more into every action of our lives, and we feel more and more the wholesome harmony of a rhythmic life. We gradually swing into rhythm with Nature through a child-like obedience to her laws.

Of one thing I must warn all nervous people who mean to try the relief to be gained from relaxation. The first effects will often be exceedingly unpleasant. The same results are apt to follow that come from the reaction after extreme excitement,—all the way from nervous nausea and giddiness to absolute fainting. This, as must be clearly seen, is a natural result from the relaxation that comes after years of habitual tension. The nerves have been held in a chronic state of excitement over something or nothing; and, of course, when their owner for the first time lets go, they begin to feel their real state, and the result of habitual strain must be unpleasant. The greater the nervous strain at the beginning, the more slowly the pupil should advance, practising in some cases only five minutes a day.

And with regard to those people who "live on their nerves," not a few, indeed very many, are so far out of the normal way of living that they detest relaxation. A hearty hatred of the relaxing motions is often met, and even when the mind is convinced of the truth of the theory, it is only with difficulty that such people can persuade themselves or be persuaded by others to work steadily at the practice until the desired result is gained.

"It makes me ten times more nervous than I was before."

"Oh, no, it does not; it only makes you realize your nervousness ten times more."

"Well, then, I do not care to realize my nervousness, it is very disagreeable."

"But, unfortunately, if you do not realize it now and relax into Nature's ways, she will knock you hard against one of her stone walls, and you will rebound with a more unpleasant realization of nervousness than is possible now."

The locomotive engine only utilizes nineteen per cent of the amount of fuel it burns, and inventors are hard at work in all directions to make an engine that will burn only the fuel needed to run it. Here is a much more valuable machine—the human engine—burning perhaps eighty-one per cent more than is needed to accomplish its ends, not through the mistake of its Divine Maker, but through the stupid, short-sighted thoughtlessness of the engineer.

Is not the economy of our vital forces of much greater importance than mechanical or business economy?

It is painful to see a man—thin and pale from the excessive nervous force he has used, and from a whole series of attacks of nervous prostration—speak with contempt of "this method of relaxation." It is not a method in any sense except that in which all the laws of Nature are methods. No one invented it, no one planned it; every one can see, who will look, that it is Nature's way and the only true way of living. To call it a new idea or method is as absurd as it would be, had we carried our tension so far as to forget sleep entirely, for some one to come with a "new method" of sleep to bring us into a normal state again; and then the people suffering most intensely from want of "tired Nature's sweet restorer" would be the most scornful in their irritation at this new idea of "sleep."

Again, there are many, especially women, who insist that they prefer the nervously excited state, and would not lose it. This is like a man's preferring to be chronically drunk. But all these abnormal states are to be expected in abnormal people, and must be quietly met by Nature's principles in order to lead the sufferers back to Nature's ways. Our minds are far enough beyond our bodies to lead us to help ourselves out of mistaken opinions; although often the sincere help of others takes us more rapidly over hard ground and prevents many a stumble.

Great nervous excitement is possible, every one knows, without muscular tension; therefore in all these motions for gaining freedom and a better physical equilibrium in nerve and muscle, the warning cannot be given too often to take every exercise easily. Do not work at it, go so far even as not to care especially whether you do it right or not, but simply do what is to be done without straining mind or body by effort. It is quite possible to make so desperate an effort to relax, that more harm than good is done. Particularly harmful is the intensity with which an effort to gain physical freedom is made by so many highly strung natures. The additional mental excitement is quite out of proportion to the gain that may come from muscular freedom. For this reason it is never advisable for one who feels the need of gaining a more natural control of nervous power to undertake the training without a teacher. If a teacher is out of the question, ten minutes practice a day is all that should be tried for several weeks.

XIII.

TRAINING FOR MOTION

"IN every new movement, in every unknown attitude needed in difficult exercises, the nerve centres have to exercise a kind of selection of the muscles, bringing into action those which favor the movement, and suppressing those which oppose it." This very evident truth Dr. Lagrange gives us in his valuable book on the Physiology of Exercise. At first, every new movement is unknown; and, owing to inherited and personal contractions, almost from the earliest movement in a child's learning to walk to the most complicated action of our daily lives, the nerve centres exercise a mistaken selection of muscles,—not only selecting more muscles than are needed for perfect co-ordination of movement, but throwing more force than necessary into the muscles selected. To a gradually increasing extent, the contracting force, instead of being withdrawn when the muscle is inactive, remains; and, as we have already seen, an arm or leg that should be passive is lifted, and the muscles are found to be contracted as if for severe action. To the surprise of the owner the contraction cannot be at once removed. Help for this habitual contraction is given in the preceding chapter. Further on Dr. Lagrange tells us that "Besides the apprenticeship of movements which are unknown, there is the improvement of already known movements." When the work of mistaken selection of muscles has gone on for years, the "improvement of already known movements," from the simplest domestic action to the accomplishment of very great purposes, is a study in itself. One must learn first to be a grown baby, and, as we have already seen, gain the exquisite passiveness of a baby; then one must learn to walk and to move by a natural process of selection, which, thanks to the contractions of his various ancestors, was not the process used for his original movements. This learning to live all over again is neither so frightful nor so difficult as it sounds. Having gained the passive state described in the last chapter, one is vastly more sensitive to unnecessary tension; and it seems often as though the child in us asserted itself, rising with alacrity to claim its right of natural movement, and with a new sense of freedom in the power gained to shun inherited and personal contractions. Certainly it is a fact that freedom of movement is gained through shunning the contractions. And this should always be kept in mind to avoid the self-consciousness and harm which come from a studied movement, not to mention the very disagreeable impression such movements give to all who appreciate their artificiality.

Motion in the human body, as well as music, is an art. An artist has very aptly said that we should so move that if every muscle struck a note, only harmony would result.

Were it so the harmony would be most exquisite, for the instrument is Nature's own. We see how far we are from a realization of natural movement when we watch carefully and note the muscular discords evident to our eyes at all times. Even the average ballet dancing, which is supposed to be the perfection of artistic movement, is merely a series of pirouettes and gymnastic contortions, with the theatrical smile of a pretty woman to throw the glare of a calcium light over the imperfections and dazzle us. The average ballet girl is not adequately trained, from the natural and artistic standpoint. If this is the case in what should be the quintessence of natural, and so of artistic movement, it is to a great degree owing to the absolute carelessness in the selection of the muscles to be used in every movement of daily life.

Many exercises which lead to the freedom of the body are well known in the letter—not in the spirit—through the so-called "Delsarte system." if they had been followed with a broad appreciation of what they were meant for and what they could lead to, before now students would have realized to a far greater extent what power is possible to the human body. But so much that is good and helpful in the "Delsarte system" has been misused, and so much of what is thoroughly artificial and unhealthy has been mixed with the useful, that one hesitates now to mention Delsarte. Either he was a wonderful genius whose thoughts and discoveries have been sadly perverted, or the inconsistencies of his teachings were great enough to limit the true power which certainly can be found in much that he has left us.

Besides the exercises already described there are many others, suited to individual needs, for gaining the freedom of each part of the body and of the body as a whole.

It is not possible to describe them clearly enough to allow them to be followed without a teacher, and to secure the desired result. Indeed, there would be danger of unpleasant results from misunderstanding. The object is so to stand that our muscles hold us, with the natural balance given them, instead of trying, as most of us do, to hold our muscles. In moving to gain this natural equilibrium we allow our muscles to carry us forward, and when they have contracted as far as is possible for one set, the antagonizing muscles carry us back. So it is with the side-to-side poising from the ankles, and the circular motion, which is a natural swinging of the muscles to find their centre of equilibrium, having once been started out of it. To stand for a moment and *think* the feet heavy is a great help in gaining the natural poising motions, but care should always be taken to hold the chest well up. Indeed, we need have no sense of effort in standing, except in raising the chest,—and that must be as if it were pulled up outside by a button in its centre, but there must be no strain in the effort.

The result of the exercises taken to free the head is shown in the power to toss the head lightly and easily, with the waist muscles, from a dropped forward to an erect position. The head shows its freedom then by the gentle swing of the neck muscles, which is entirely involuntary and comes from the impetus given them in tossing the head.

Tension in the muscles of the neck is often very difficult to overcome; because, among other reasons, the sensations coming from certain forms of nervous over-strain are very commonly referred to the region of the base of the brain. It is not unusual to find the back of the neck rigid in extreme tension, and whether the strain is very severe or not, great care must be taken to free it by slow degrees, and the motions should at first be practised only a few minutes at a time. I can hardly warn readers too often against the possibility of an unpleasant reaction, if the relaxing is practised too long, or gained too rapidly.

Then should come exercises for freeing the arms; and these can be taken sitting. Let the arms hang heavily at the sides; raise one arm slowly, feeling the weight more and more distinctly, and only contracting the shoulder muscles. It is well to raise it a few inches, then drop it heavily and try again,—each time taking force out of the lower muscles by thinking the arm heavy, and the motive power in the shoulder. If the arm itself can rest heavily on some one's hand while you are still raising it from the shoulder, that proves that you have succeeded in withdrawing the useless tension. Most arms feel stiff all the way along, when the owners raise them. Your arm must be raised until high overhead, the hand hanging from the wrist and dropped into your lap or down at the side, letting the elbow "give," so that the upper arm drops first, and then the fore arm and hand,— like three heavy sand-bags sewed together. The arm can be brought up to the level of the shoulder, and then round in front and dropped. To prove its freedom, toss it with the shoulder muscles from the side into the lap. Watch carefully that the arm itself has no more tension than if it were a sand-bag hung at the side, and could only be moved by the shoulder. After practising this two or three times so that the arms are relaxed enough to make you more sensitive to tension, one hundred times a day you will find your arms held rigidly, while you are listening or talking or walking. Every day you will grow more sensitive to the useless tension, and every day gain new power to drop it. This is wherein the real practice comes. An hour or two hours a day of relaxing exercises will amount to nothing if at the same time we are not careful to use the freedom gained, and to do everything more naturally. It is often said, "But I cannot waste time watching all day to see if I am using too much force." There is no need to watch; having once started in the right direction, if you drop useless muscular contraction every time you notice it, that is enough. It will be as natural to do that as for a musician to correct a discord which he has inadvertently made on the piano.

There are no motions so quieting, so helpful in the general freeing of the body, as the motions of the spine. There are no motions more difficult to describe, or which should be more carefully directed. The habitual rigidity of the spine, as compared with its possible freedom, is more noticeable in training, of course, than is that of any other part of the body. Each vertebra should be so distinctly independent of every other, as to make the spine as smoothly jointed as the toy snakes, which, when we hold the tip of the tail in our fingers, curve in all directions. Most of us have spinal columns that more or less resemble ramrods. It is a surprise and delight to find what can be accomplished, when the muscles of the spine and back are free and under control. Of course the natural state of the spine, as the seat of a great nervous centre, affects many muscles of the body, and, on the other hand, the freedom of these muscles reacts favorably upon the spine.

The legs are freed for standing and walking by shaking the foot free from the ankle with the leg, swinging the fore leg from the upper leg, and so freeing the muscles at the knee, and by standing on a footstool and letting one leg hang off the stool a dead weight while swinging it round from the hip. Greater freedom and ease of movement can be gained by standing on the floor and swinging the leg from the hip as high as possible. Be sure that the only effort for motion is in the muscles of the hip. There are innumerable other motions to free the legs, and often a great variety must be practised before the freedom can be gained.

The muscles of the chest and waist are freed through a series of motions, the result of which is shown in the ability to toss the body lightly from the hips, as the head is tossed from the waist muscles; and there follows the same gentle involuntary swing of the muscles of the waist which surprises one so pleasantly in the neck muscles after tossing the head, and gives a new realization of what physical freedom is.

In tossing the body the motion must be successive, like running the scale with the vertebrae.

In no motion should the muscles work *en masse*. The more perfect the co-ordination of muscles in any movement, the more truly each muscle holds its own individuality. This power of freedom in motion should be worked for after once approaching the natural equilibrium. If you rest on your left leg, it pushes your left hip a little farther out, which causes your body to swerve slightly to the right,—and, to keep the balance true, the head again tips to the left a little. Now rise slowly and freely from that to standing on both feet, with body and head erect; then drop on the right foot with the body to left, and head to right. Here again, as in the motions with the spine, there is a great difference in the way they are practised. Their main object is to help the muscles to an independent individual co-ordination, and there should be a new sense of ease and freedom every time we practise it. Hold the chest up, and push yourself erect with the ball of your free foot. The more the weight is thought into the feet the freer the muscles are for action, provided the chest is well raised. The forward and back spinal motion should be taken standing also; and there is a gentle circular motion of the entire body which proves the freedom of all the muscles for natural movement, and is most restful in its result.

The study for free movement in the arms and legs should of course be separate. The law that every part moves from something prior to it, is illustrated exquisitely in the motion of the fingers from the wrist. Here also the individuality of the muscles in their perfect co-ordination is pleasantly illustrated. To gain ease of movement in the fore arm, its motive power must seem to be in the upper arm; the motive power for the entire arm must seem to be centred in the shoulder. When through various exercises a natural co-ordination of the muscles is gained, the arm can be moved in curves from the shoulder, which remind one of a graceful snake; and the balance is so true that the motion seems hardly more than a thought in the amount of effort it takes. Great care should be given to freeing the hands and fingers. Because the hand is in such constant communication with the brain, the tension of the entire body often seems to be reflected there. Sometimes it is even necessary to train the hand to some extent in the earliest lessons.

Exercises for movement in the legs are to free the joints, so that motions may follow one another as in the arm,—the foot from the ankle; the lower leg from the upper leg; the upper leg from the hip; and, as—in the arm, the free action of the joints in the leg comes as we seem to centre the motive power in the hip. There is then the same grace and ease of movement which we gain in the arm, simply because the muscles have their natural equilibrium.

Thus the motive power of the body will seem to be gradually drawn to an imaginary centre in the lower part of the trunk,—which simply means withdrawing superfluous tension from every part. The exercise to help establish this equilibrium is graceful, and not difficult if we take it quietly and easily, using the mind to hold a balance without effort. Raise the right arm diagonally forward, the left leg diagonally back,—the arm must be high up, the foot just off the floor, so that as far as possible you make a direct line from the wrist to the ankle; in this attitude stretch all muscles across the body from left to right slowly and steadily, then relax quite as slowly. Now, be sure your arm and leg are free from all tension, and swing them very slowly, as if they were one piece, to as nearly a horizontal position as they can reach; then slowly pivot round until you bring your arm diagonally back and your leg diagonally forward; still horizontal, pivot again to the starting point; then bring leg down and arm up, always keeping them as in a line, until your foot is again off the floor; then slowly lower your arm and let your foot rest on the floor so that gradually your whole weight rests on that leg, and the other is free to swing up and pivot with the opposite arm. All this must be done slowly and without strain of any kind. The motions which follow in sets are for the better daily working of the body, as well as to establish its freedom. The first set is called the "Big Rhythms," because it takes mainly the rhythmic movement of the larger muscles of the body, and is meant, through movements taken on one foot, to give a true balance in the poise of the body as well as to make habitual the natural co-ordination in the action of all the larger muscles. It is like practising a series of big musical chords to accustom our ears to their harmonies. The second set, named the "Little Rhythms,"—because that is a convenient way of designating it,—is a series meant to include the movement of all the smaller muscles as well as the large ones, and is carried out even to the fingers. The third set is for spring and rapid motion, especially in joints of arms and legs.

Of course having once found the body's natural freedom, the variety of motions is as great as the variety of musical sounds and combinations possible to an instrument which will respond to every tone in the musical scale. It is in opening the way for this natural motion that the exquisite possibilities in motion purely artistic dawn upon us with ever-increasing light. And as in music it is the sonata, the waltz, or the nocturne we must feel, not the mechanical process of our own performance,—so in moving, it is the beautiful, natural harmonies of the muscles, from the big rhythms to all the smaller ones, that we must feel and make others feel, and not the mere mechanical grace of our bodies; and we can move a sonata from the first to the last, changing the time and holding the theme so that the soul will be touched through the eye, as it is through the ear now in music. But, according to the present state of the human body, more than one generation will pass before we reach, or know the beginning of, the highest artistic power of motion. If art is Nature illuminated, one must have some slight appreciation and experience of Nature before attempting her illumination.

The set of motions mentioned can be only very inadequately described in print. But although they are graceful, because they are natural, the first idea in practising them is that they are a means to an end, not an end in themselves. For in the big and little rhythms and the springing motions, in practising them over and over again we are establishing the habit of natural motion, and will carry it more and more into everything we do.

If the work of the brain in muscular exercise were reduced to its minimum, the consequent benefit from all exercise would greatly increase.

A new movement can be learned with facility in proportion to the power for dropping at the time all impressions of previous movements. In training to take every motion easily, after a time the brain-work is relieved, for we move with ease,—that is, with a natural co-ordination of muscles, automatically,—in every known motion; and we lessen very greatly the mental strain, in learning a new movement, by gaining the power to relax entirely at first, and then, out of a free body, choose the muscles needed, and so avoid the nervous strain of useless muscular experiment.

So far as the mere muscular movement goes, the sensation is that of being well oiled. As for instance, in a natural walk, where the swinging muscles and the standing muscles act and rest in alternate rhythmic action, the chest is held high, the side muscles free to move in, harmony with the legs, and all the spring in the body brought into play through inclining slightly forward and pushing with the ball of the back foot, the arms swinging naturally without tension. Walking with a free body is often one of the best forms of rest, and in the varying forms of motion arranged for practice we are enabled to realize, that "perfect harmony of action in the entire man invigorates every part."

XIV.

MIND TRAINING

IT will be plainly seen that this training of the body is at the same time a training of the mind, and indeed it is in essence a training of the will. For as we think of it carefully and analyze it to its fundamental principles, we realize that it might almost be summed up as in itself a training of the will alone. That is certainly what it leads to, and where it leads from.

Maudsley tells us that "he who is incapable of guiding his muscles, is incapable of concentrating his mind;" and it would seem to follow, by a natural sequence, that training for the best use of all the powers given us should begin with the muscles, and continue through the nerves and the senses to the mind,—all by means of the will, which should gradually remove all personal contractions and obstructions to the wholesome working of the law of cause and effect.

Help a child to use his own ability of gaining free muscles, nerves clear to take impressions through every sense, a mind open to recognize them, and a will alive with interest in and love for finding the best in each new sensation or truth, and what can he not reach in power of use to others and in his own growth.

The consistency of creation is perfect. The law that applies to the guidance of the muscles works just as truly in training the senses and the mind.

A new movement can be learned with facility in proportion to the power of dropping at the time all impressions of previous movements. Quickness and keenness of sense are gained only in proportion to the power of quieting the senses not in use, and erasing previous impressions upon the sense which is active at the time.

True concentration of mind means the ability to drop every subject but that centred upon. Tell one man to concentrate his mind on a difficult problem until he has worked it out,—he will clinch his fists, tighten his throat, hold his teeth hard together, and contract nobody knows how many more muscles in his body, burning and wasting fuel in a hundred or more places where it should be saved. This is *not* concentration. Concentration means the focussing of a force; and when the mathematical faculty of the brain alone should be at work, the force is not focussed if it is at the same time flying over all other parts of the body in useless strain of innumerable muscles. Tell another man, one who works naturally, to solve the same problem,—he will instinctively and at once "erase all previous impressions" in muscle and nerve, and with a quiet, earnest expression, not a face knotted with useless strain, will concentrate upon his work. The result, so far as the problem itself is concerned, may be the same in both cases; but the result upon the physique of the men who have undertaken the work will be vastly different.

It will be insisted upon by many, and, strange as it may seem, by many who have a large share of good sense, that they can work better with this extra tension. "For," the explanation is, "it is natural to me." That may be, but it is not natural to Nature; and however difficult it may be at first to drop our own way and adopt Nature's, the proportionate gain is very great in the end.

Normal exercise often stimulates the brain, and by promoting more vigorous circulation, and so greater physical activity all over the body, helps the brain to work more easily. Therefore some men can think better while walking.

This is quite unlike the superfluous strain of nervous motion, which, however it may seem to help at the time, eventually and steadily lessens mental power instead of increasing it. The distinction between motion which wholesomely increases the brain activity and that which is simply unnecessary tension, is not difficult to discern when our eyes are well opened to superfluous effort. This misdirected force seems to be the secret of much of the overwork in schools, and the consequent physical breakdown of school children, especially girls. It is not that they have too much to do, it is that they do not know how to study naturally, and with the real concentration which learns the lesson most quickly, most surely, and with the least amount of effort. They study a lesson with all the muscles of the body when only the brain is needed, with a running accompaniment of worry for fear it will not be learned.

Girls can be, have been, trained out of worrying about their lessons. Nervous strain is often extreme in students, from lesson-worry alone; and indeed in many cases it is the worry that tires and brings illness, and not the study. Worry is brain tension. It is partly a vague, unformed sense that work is not being done in the best way which makes the pressure more than it need be; and instead of quietly studying to work to better advantage, the worrier allows herself to get more and more oppressed by her anxieties,— as we have seen a child grow cross over a snarl of twine which, with very little patience, might be easily unravelled, but in which, in the child's nervous annoyance, every knot is pulled tighter. Perhaps we ought hardly to expect as much from the worried student as from the child, because the ideas of how to study arc so vague that they seldom bring a realization of the fact that there might be an improvement in the way of studying.

This possible improvement may be easily shown. I have taken a girl inclined to the mistaken way of working, asked her to lie on the floor where she could give up entirely to the force of gravity,—then after helping her to a certain amount of passivity, so that at least she looked quiet, have asked her to give me a list of her lessons. Before opening her mouth to answer, she moved in little nervous twitches, apparently every muscle in her body, from head to foot. I stopped her, took time to bring her again to a quiet state, and then repeated the question. Again the nervous movement began, but this time the child exclaimed, "Why, isn't it funny? I cannot think without moving all over!" Here was the Rubicon crossed. She had become alive to her own superfluous tension; and after that to train her not only to think without moving all over, but to answer questions easily and quietly and so with more expression, and then to study with greatly decreased effort, was a very pleasant process.

Every boy and girl should have this training to a greater or less degree. It is a steady, regular process, and should be so taken. We have come through too many generations of misused force to get back into a natural use of our powers in any rapid way; it must come step by step, as a man is trained to use a complicated machine. It seems hardly fair to compare such training to the use of a machine,—it opens to us such extensive and unlimited power. We can only make the comparison with regard to the first process of development.

A training for concentration of mind should begin with the muscles. First, learn to withdraw the will from the muscles entirely. Learn, next, to direct the will over the muscles of one arm while the rest of the body is perfectly free and relaxed,—first, by stretching the arm slowly and steadily, and then allowing it to relax; next, by clinching the fist and drawing the arm up with all the force possible until the elbow is entirely bent. There is not one person in ten, hardly one in a hundred, who can command his muscles to that slight extent. At first some one must lift the arm that should be free, and drop it several times while the muscles of the other arm are contracting; that will make the unnecessary tension evident. There are also ways by which the free arm can be tested without the help of a second person.

The power of directing the will over various muscles that should be independent, without the so-called sympathetic contraction of other muscles, should be gained all over the body. This is the beginning of concentration in a true sense of the word. The necessity for returning to an absolute freedom of body before directing the will to any new part cannot be too often impressed upon the mind. Having once "sensed" a free body—so to speak—we are not masters until we gain the power to return to it at a moment's notice. In a second we can "erase previous impressions" for the time; and that is the foundation, the rock, upon which our house is built.

Then follows the process of learning to think and to speak in freedom. First, as to useless muscular contractions. Watch children work their hands when reciting in class. Tell them to stop, and the poor things will, with great effort, hold their hands rigidly still, and suffer from the discomfort and strain of doing so. Help them to freedom of body, then to the sense that the working of their hands is not really needed, and they will learn to recite with a feeling of freedom which is better than they can understand. Sometimes a child must be put on the floor to learn to think quietly and directly, and to follow the same directions in this manner of answering. It would be better if this could always be done with thoughtful care and watching; but as this would be inappropriate with large classes, there are quieting and relaxing exercises to be practised sitting and standing, which will bring children to a normal freedom, and help them to drop muscular contractions which interfere with ease and control of thought and expression. Pictures can be described,—scenes from Shakespeare, for instance,—in the child's own words, while making quiet motions. Such exercise increases the sensitiveness to muscular contraction, and unnecessary muscular contraction, beside something to avoid in itself, obviously makes thought *indirect.* A child must think quietly, to express his thought quietly and directly. This exercise, of course, also cultivates the imagination.

In all this work, as clear channels are opened for impression and expression, the faculties themselves naturally have a freer growth. The process of quiet thought and expression must be trained in all phases,—from the slow description of something seen or imagined or remembered, to the quick and correct answer required to an example in mental arithmetic, or any other rapid thinking. This, of course, means a growth in power of attention,— attention which is real concentration, not the strained attention habitual to most of us, and which being abnormal in itself causes abnormal reaction. And this natural attention is learned in the use of each separate sense,—to see, to hear, to taste, to smell, to touch with quick and exact impression and immediate expression, if required, and a in obedience to the natural law of the conservation of human energy.

With the power of studying freely, comes that of dropping a lesson when it is once well learned, and finding it ready when needed for recitation or for any other use. The temptation to take our work into our play is very great, and often cannot be overcome until we have learned how to "erase all previous impressions." The concentration which enables us all through life to be intent upon the one thing we are doing, whether it is tennis or trigonometry, and drop what we have in hand at once and entirely at the right time, free to give out attention fully to the next duty or pleasure, is our saving health in mind and body. The trouble is we are afraid. We have no trust. A child is afraid to stop thinking of a lesson after it is learned,—afraid he will forget it. When he has once been persuaded to drop it, the surprise when he takes it up again, to find it more clearly impressed upon his mind, is delightful. One must trust to the digestion of a lesson, as to that of a good wholesome dinner. Worry and anxiety interfere with the one as much as with the other. If you can drop a muscle when you have ceased using it, that leads to the power of dropping a subject in mind; as the muscle is fresher for use when you need it, so the subject seems to have grown in you, and your grasp seems to be stronger when you recur to it.

The law of rhythm must be carefully followed in this training for the use of the mind. Do not study too long at a time. It makes a natural reaction impossible. Arrange the work so that lessons as far unlike as possible may be studied in immediate succession. We help to the healthy reaction of one faculty, by exercising another that is quite different.

This principle should be inculcated in classes, and for that purpose a regular programme of class work should be followed, calculated to bring about the best results in all branches of study.

The first care should be to gain quiet, as through repose of mind and body we cultivate the power to "erase all previous impressions." In class, quiet, rhythmic breathing, with closed eyes, is most helpful for a beginning. The eyes must be closed and opened slowly and gently, not snapped together or apart; and fifty breaths, a little longer than they would naturally be, are enough to quiet a class. The breaths must be counted, to keep the mind from wandering, and the faces must be watched very carefully, for the expression often shows anything but quiet. For this reason it is necessary, in initiating a class, to begin with simple relaxing motions; later these motions will follow the breathing. Then follow exercises for directing the muscles. The force is directed into one arm with the rest of the body free, and so in various simple exercises the power of directing the will only to the muscles needed is cultivated. After the muscle-work, the pupils are asked to centre their minds for a minute on one subject,—the subject to be chosen by some member, with slight help to lead the choice to something that will be suggestive for a minute's thinking. At first it seems impossible to hold one subject in mind for a minute; but the power grows rapidly as we learn the natural way of concentrating, and instead of trying to hold on to our subject, allow the subject to hold us by refusing entrance to every other thought. In the latter case one suggestion follows another with an ease and pleasantness which reminds one of walking through new paths and seeing on every side something fresh and unexpected. Then the class is asked to think of a list of flowers, trees, countries, authors, painters, or whatever may be suggested, and see who can think of the greatest number in one minute. At first, the mind will trip and creak and hesitate over the work, but with practice the list comes steadily and easily. Then follow exercises for quickness and exactness of sight, then for hearing, and finally for the memory. All through this process, by constant help and suggestion, the pupils are brought to the natural concentration. With regard to the memory, especial care should be taken, for the harm done by a mechanical training of the memory can hardly be computed. Repose and the consequent freedom of body and mind lead to an opening of all the faculties for better use; if that is so, a teacher must be more than ever alive to lead pupils to the spirit of all they are to learn, and make the letter in every sense suggestive of the spirit. First, care should be taken to give something worth memorizing; secondly, ideas must be memorized before the words. A word is a symbol, and in so far as we have the habit of regarding it as such, will each word we hear be more and more suggestive to us. With this habit well cultivated, one sees more in a single glance at a poem than many could see in several readings. Yet the reader who sees the most may be unable to repeat the poem word for word. In cultivating the memory, the training should be first for the attention, then for the imagination and the power of suggestive thought; and from the opening of these faculties a true memory will grow. The mechanical power of repeating after once hearing so many words is a thing in itself to be dreaded. Let the pupil first see in mind a series of pictures as the poem or page is read, then describe them in his own words, and if the words of the author are well worth remembering the pupil should be led to them from the ideas. In the same way a series of interesting or helpful thoughts can be learned.

Avoidance of mere mechanism cannot be too strongly insisted upon; for exercise for attaining a wholesome, natural guidance of mind and body cannot be successful unless it rouses in the mind an appreciation of the laws of Nature which we are bound to obey. A conscious experience of the results of such obedience is essential to growth.

XV.

ARTISTIC CONSIDERATIONS

ALTHOUGH so much time and care are given to the various means of artistic expression, it is a singular fact that comparatively little attention is given to the use of the very first instrument which should be under command before any secondary instrument can be made perfectly expressive.

An old artist who thanked his friend for admiring his pictures added: "If you could only see the pictures in my brain. But—" pointing to his brain and then to the ends of his fingers—"the channels from here to here are so long!" The very sad tone which we can hear in the wail of the painter expresses strongly the deficiencies of our age in all its artistic efforts. The channels are shorter just in proportion to their openness. If the way from the brain to the ends of the fingers is perfectly clear, the brain can guide the ends of the fingers to carry out truly its own aspirations, and the honest expression of the brain will lead always to higher ideals. But the channels cannot be free, and the artist will be bound so long as there is superfluous tension in any part of the body. So absolutely necessary, is it for the best artistic expression that the body should throughout be only a servant of the mind, that the more we think of it the more singular it seems that the training of the body to a childlike state is not regarded as essential, and taken as a matter of course, even as we take our regular nourishment.

The artificial is tension in its many trying and disagreeable phases. Art is freedom, equilibrium, rhythm,— anything and everything that means wholesome life and growth toward all that is really the good, the true, and the beautiful.

Art is immeasurably greater than we are. If we are free and quiet, the poem, the music, the picture will carry us, so that we shall be surprised at our own expression; and when we have finished, instead of being personally elated with conceited delight in what we have done, or exhausted with the superfluous effort used, we shall feel as if a strong wind had blown through us and cleared us for better work in the future.

Every genius obeys the true principle. It is because a genius is involuntarily under the law of his art that he is pervaded by its power. But we who have only talent must learn the laws of genius, which are the laws of Nature, and by careful study and steady practice in shunning all personal obstructions to the laws, bring ourselves under their sway.

Who would wish to play on a stringed instrument already vibrating with the touch of some one else, or even with the last touch we ourselves gave it. What noise, what discord, with no possible harmonies! So it is with our nerves and muscles. They cannot be used for artistic purposes to the height of their best powers while they are tense and vibrating to our own personal states or habits; so that the first thing is to free them absolutely, and not only keep them free by constant practice, but so train them that they will become perfectly free at a moment's notice, and ready to respond clearly to whatever the heart and the mind want to express.

The finer the instrument, the lighter the touch it will vibrate to. Indeed it must have a light touch to respond clearly with musical harmonies; any other touch would blur. With a fine piano or a violin, whether the effect is to be *piano* or *fortissimo,* the touch should be only with the amount of force needed to give a clear vibration, and the ease with which a fortissimo effect is thus produced is astonishing. It is only those with the most delicate touch who can produce from a fine piano grand and powerful harmonies without a blur.

The response in a human instrument to a really light touch is far more wonderful than that from any instrument made by man; and bodily effort blurs just as much more in proportion. The muscles are all so exquisitely balanced in their power for co-ordinate movement, that a muscle pulling one way is almost entirely freed from effort by the equalizing power of the antagonizing muscle; and at some rare moments when we have really found the equilibrium and can keep it, we seem to do no more than *think* a movement or a tone or a combination of words, and they come with so slight a physical exertion that it seems like no effort at all.

So far are we from our possibilities in this lightness of touch in the use of our bodies, that it is impossible now for most of us to touch as lightly as would, after training, bring the most powerful response. One of the best laws for artistic practice is, "Every day less effort, every day more power." As the art of acting is the only art where the whole body is used with no subordinate instrument, let us look at that with regard to the best results to be obtained by means of relief from superfluous tension. The effects of unnecessary effort are strongly felt in the exhaustion which follows the interpretation of a very exciting role. It is a law without exception, that if I absorb an emotion and allow my own nerves to be shaken by it, I fail to give it in all its expressive power to the audience; and not only do I fall far short in my artistic interpretation, but because of that very failure, come off the stage with just so much nervous force wasted. Certain as this law is, and infallible as are its effects, it is not only generally disbelieved, but it is seldom thought of at all. I must feet Juliet in my heart, understand her with my mind, and let her vibrate clearly *across* my nerves, to the audience. The moment I let my nerves be shaken as Juliet's nerves were in reality, I am absorbing her myself, misusing nervous force, preparing to come off the stage thoroughly exhausted, and keeping her away from the audience. The present low state of the drama is largely due to this failure to recognize and practise a natural use of the nervous force. To work up an emotion, a most pernicious practice followed by young aspirants, means to work your nerves up to a state of mild or even severe hysteria. This morbid, inartistic, nervous excitement actually trains men and women to the loss of all emotional control, and no wonder that their nerves play the mischief with them, and that the atmosphere of the stage is kept in its present murkiness. The power to work the nerves up in the beginning finally carries them to the state where they must be more artificially urged by stimulants; and when the actor is off the stage he has no self-control at all. This all means misused and over-used force. In no schools is the general influence so absolutely morbid and unwholesome, as in most of the schools of elocution and acting.

The methods by which the necessity for artificial stimulants can be overcome are so simple and so pleasant and so immediately effective, that it is worth taking the time and space to describe them briefly. Of course, to begin with, the body must be trained to perfect freedom in repose, and then to freedom in its use. A very simple way of practising is to take the most relaxed attitude possible, and then, without changing it, to recite *with all the expression that belongs to it* some poem or selection from a play full of emotional power. You will become sensitive at once to any new tension, and must stop and drop it. At first, an hour's daily practice will be merely a beginning over and over,—

the nervous tension will be so evident,—but the final reward is well worth working and waiting for.

It is well to begin by simply inhaling through the nose, and exhaling quietly through the mouth several times; then inhale and exhale an exclamation in every form of feeling you can think of Let the exclamation come as easily and freely as the breath alone, without superfluous tension in any part of the body. So much freedom gained, inhale as before, and exhale brief expressive sentences,—beginning with very simple expressions, and taking sentences that express more and more feeling as your freedom is better established. This practice can be continued until you are able to recite the potion scene in Juliet, or any of Lady Macbeth's most powerful speeches, with an case and freedom which is surprising. This refers only to the voice; the practice which has been spoken of in a previous chapter brings the same effect in gesture.

It will be readily seen that this power once gained, no actor would find it necessary to skip every other night, in consequence of the severe fatigue which follows the acting of an emotional role. Not only is the physical fatigue saved, but the power of expression, the power for intense acting, so far as it impresses the audience, is steadily increased.

The inability of young persons to express an emotion which they feel and appreciate heartily, can be always overcome in this way. Relaxing frees the channels, and the channels being open the real poetic or dramatic feeling cannot be held back. The relief is as if one were let out of prison. Personal faults that come from self-consciousness and nervous tension may be often cured entirely without the necessity of drawing attention to them, simply by relaxing.

Dramatic instinct is a delicate perception of, quick and keen sympathies for, and ability to express the various phases of human nature. Deep study and care are necessary for the best development of these faculties; but the nerves must be left free to be guided to the true expression,— neither allowed to vibrate to the ecstatic delight of the impressions, or in mistaken sympathy with them, but kept clear as conductors of all the heart can feel and the mind understand in the character or poem to be interpreted.

This may sound cold. It is not; it is merely a process of relieving superfluous nervous tension in acting, by which obstructions are removed so that real sympathetic emotions can be stronger and fuller, and perceptions keener. Those who get no farther than emotional vibrations of the nerves in acting, know nothing whatever of the greatness or power of true dramatic instinct.

There are three distinct schools of dramatic art,—one may be called dramatic hysteria, the second dramatic hypocrisy. The first means emotional excitement and nervous exhaustion; the second artificial simulation of a feeling. Dramatic sincerity is the third school, and the school that seems most truly artistic. What a wonderful training is that which might,—which ought to be given an actor to help him rise to the highest possibility of his art!

A free body, exquisitely responsive to every command of the mind, is absolutely necessary; therefore there should be a perfect physical training. A quick and keen perception to appreciate noble thoughts, holding each idea distinctly, and knowing the relations of each idea to the others, must certainly be cultivated; for in acting, every idea, every word, should come clearly, each taking its own place in the thought expressed.

Broad human sympathies, the imaginative power of identifying himself with all phases of human nature, if he has an ideal in his profession above the average, an actor cannot lack. This last is quite impossible without broad human charity; for "to observe truly you must sympathize with those you observe, and to sympathize with them you must love them, and to love them you must forget yourself." And all these requisites—the physical state, the understanding, and the large heart—seem to centre in the expression of a well-trained voice,—a voice in which there is the minimum of body and the maximum of soul.

By training, I always mean a training into Nature. As I have said before, if art is Nature illuminated, we must find Nature before we can reach art. The trouble is that in acting, more than in any other art, the distinction between what is artistic and what is artificial is neither clearly understood nor appreciated; yet so marked is the difference when once we see it, that the artificial may well be called the hell of art, as art itself is heavenly.

Sincerity and simplicity are the foundations of art. A feigning of either is often necessary to the artificial, but many times impossible. Although the external effect of this natural training is a great saving of nervous force in acting, the height of its power cannot be reached except through a simple aim, from the very heart, toward sincere artistic expression.

So much for acting. It is a magnificent study, and should be more truly wholesome in its effects than any other art, because it deals with the entire body. But, alas I it seems now the most thoroughly morbid and unwholesome.

All that has been said of acting will apply also to singing, especially to dramatic singing and study for opera; only with singing even more care should be taken. No singer realizes the necessity of a quiet, absolutely free body for the best expression of a high note, until having gained a certain physical freedom without singing, she takes a high note and is made sensitive to the superfluous tension all over the body, and later learns to reach the same note with the repose which is natural; then the contrast between the natural and the unnatural methods of singing becomes most evident,— and not with high notes alone, but with all notes, and all combinations of notes. I speak of the high note first, because that is an extreme; for with the majority of singers there is always more or less fear when a high note is coming lest it may not be reached easily and with all the clearness that belongs to it. This fear in itself is tension. For that reason one must learn to relax to a high note. A free body relieves the singer immensely from the mechanism of singing. So perfect is the unity of the body that a voice will not obey perfectly unless the body, as a whole, be free. Once secure in the freedom of voice and body to obey, the song can burst forth with all the musical feeling, and all the deep appreciation of the words of which the singer is capable. Now, unfortunately, it is not unusual in listening to a public singer, to feel keenly that he is entirely adsorbed in the mechanism of his art.

If this freedom is so helpful, indeed so necessary, to reach one's highest power in singing, it is absolutely essential on the operatic stage. With it we should have less of the wooden motion so common to singers in opera. When one is free, physically free, the music seems to draw out the acting. With a great composer and an interpreter free to respond, the music and the body of the actor are one in their power of expressing the emotions. And the songs without words of the interludes so affect the spirit of the singer that, whether quiet or in motion, he seems, through being a living embodiment of the music, to impress the sense of seeing so that it increases the pleasure of hearing.

I am aware that this standard is ideal; but it is not impossible to approach it,—to come at least much nearer to it than we do now, when the physical movements on the stage are such, that one wants to listen to most operas with closed eyes.

We have considered artistic expression when the human body alone is the instrument. When the body is merely a means to the use of a secondary instrument, a primary training of the body itself is equally necessary.

A pianist practises for hours to command his fingers and gain a touch which will bring the soul from his music, without in the least realizing that so long as he is keeping other muscles in his body tense, and allowing the nervous force to expend itself unnecessarily in other directions, there never will be clear and open channels from his brain to his fingers; and as he literally plays with his brain, and not with his fingers, free channels for a magnetic touch are indispensable.

To watch a body *give* to the rhythm of the music in playing is most fascinating. Although the motion is slight, the contrast between that and a pianist stiff and rigid with superfluous tension is, very marked, and the difference in touch when one relaxes to the music with free channels has been very clearly proved. Beside this, the freedom in mechanism which follows the exercises for arms and hands is strikingly noticeable.

With the violin, the same physical equilibrium of motion must be gained; in fact it is equally necessary in all musical performance, as the perfect freedom of the body is always necessary before it can reach its highest power in the use of any secondary instrument.

In painting, the freer a body is the more perfectly the mind can direct it. How often we can see clearly in our minds a straight line or a curve or a combination of both, but our hands will not obey the brain, and the picture fails. It does not by any means follow that with free bodies we can direct the hand at once to whatever the brain desires, but simply that by making the body free, and so a perfect servant of the mind, it can be brought to obey the mind in a much shorter time and more directly, and so become a truer channel for whatever the mind wishes to accomplish.

In the highest art, whatever form it may take, the law of simplicity is perfectly illustrated.

It would be tiresome to go through a list of the various forms of artistic expression; enough has been said to show the necessity for a free body, sensitive to respond to, quick to obey, and open to express the commands of its owner.

XVI.

TESTS

ADOPTING the phrase of our forefathers, with all its force and brevity, we say, "The proof of the pudding is in the eating."

If the laws adduced in this book are Nature's laws, they should preserve us in health and strength. And so they do just so far as we truly and fully obey them.

Then are students and teachers of these laws never ill, never run down, "nervous," or prostrated? Yes, they are sometimes ill, sometimes run down and overworked, and suffer the many evil effects ensuing; but the work which has produced these results is much greater and more laborious than would have been possible without the practice of the principles. At the same time their states of illness occur because they only partially obey the laws. In the degree which they obey they will be preserved from the effects of tensity, overstrung nerves, and generally worn-out bodies; and in sickness coming from other causes—mechanical, hereditary, etc.—again, according to their obedience, they will be held in all possible physical and mental peace, so that the disease may wither and drop like the decayed leaf of a plant.

As well might we ask of the wisest clergyman in the land, Do his truths *never* fail him? Is he *always* held in harmony and nobility by their power? However great and good the man may be, this state of perfection will never be reached in this world.

In exact parallel to the spiritual laws upon which all universal truth, of all religions, is founded, are the truths of this teaching of physical peace and equilibrium. As religion applies to all the needs of the soul, so this applies to all the needs of the body. As a man may be continually progressing in nobility of thought and action, and yet find himself under peculiar circumstances tried even to the stumbling point,— so may the student of bodily quiet and equilibrium, who appears even to a very careful observer to be in surprising possession of his forces, under a similar test stumble and fall into some form of the evil effects out of which he has had power to lead others.

It is important that this parallelism should be recognized, that the unity of these truths may be finally accomplished in the living; therefore we repeat, Is this any more possible than that the full control of the soul should be at once possessed?

Think of the marvellous construction of the human body,—the exquisite adjustment of its economy. Could a power of control sufficient to apply to its every detail be fully acquired at once, or even in a life-time?

But when one does fall who has made himself even partially at one with Nature's way of living, the power of patient waiting for relief is very different. He separates himself from his ailments in a way which without the preparation would be to him unknown. He has, without drug or other external assistance, an anodyne always within himself which he can use at pleasure. He positively experiences that "underneath are the everlasting arms," and the power to experience this gives him much respite from pain.

Pain is so often prolonged and accentuated *by dwelling in its memory,* living in a self-pity of the time when it shall come again! The patient who comes to his test with the bodily and mental repose already acquired, cuts off each day from the last, each hour from the last, one might almost say each breath from the last, so strong is his confidence in the renewal of forces possible to those who give themselves quite trustfully into Nature's hands.

It is not that they refuse external aid or precaution. No; indeed the very quiet within makes them feel most keenly when it is orderly to rest and seek the advice of others. Also it makes them faithful in following every direction which will take them back into the rhythm of a healthful life.

But while they do this they do not centre upon it. They take the precautions as a means and not as an end. They centre upon that which they have within themselves, and they know that that possible power being in a state of disorder and chaos no one or all of the outside measures are of any value.

As patients prepared by the work return into normal life, the false exhilaration, which is a sure sign of another stumble, is seen and avoided. They have learned a serious lesson in economy, and they profit by it. Where they were free before, they become more so; and where they were not, they quietly set themselves toward constant gain. They work at lower pressure, steadily gaining in spreading the freedom and quiet deeper into their systems, thus lessening the danger of future falls.

Let us state some of the causes for "breaking down," even while trying well to learn Nature's ways.

First, a trust in one's own capacity for freedom and quiet. "I can do this, now that I know how to relax." When truly considered, the thing is out of reason, and we should say, "Because I know how to relax, I see that I must not do this."

The case is the same with the gymnast who greatly overtaxes his muscle, having foolishly concluded that because he has had some training he can successfully meet the test. There is nothing so truly stupid as self-satisfaction; and these errors, with all others of the same nature, re fruits of our stupidity, and unless shunned surely lead us into trouble.

Some natures, after practice, relax so easily that they are soon met by the dangers of overrelaxation. Let them remember that it is really equilibrium they are seeking, and

111

by balancing their activity and their relaxation, and relaxing only as a means to an end,—the end of greater activity and use later,—they avoid any such ill effect.

As the gymnast can mistake the purpose of his muscular development, putting it in the place of greater things, regarding it as an end instead of a means,—so can he who is training for a better use of his nervous force. In the latter case, the signs of this error are a slackened circulation, a loathing to activity, and various evanescent sensations of peace and satisfaction which bear no test, vanishing as soon as they are brought to the slightest trial.

Unless you take up your work with fresh interest and renewed vigor each time after practice, you may know that all is not as it should be.

To avoid all these mistakes, examine the work of each day and let the next improve upon it.

If you are in great need of relaxing, take more exercise in the fresh air. If unable to exercise, get your balance by using slow and steady breaths, which push the blood vigorously over its path in the body, and give one, to a degree, the effect of exercise.

Do not mistake the disorders which come at first, when turning away from an unnatural and wasteful life of contractions, for the effects of relaxing. Such disorders are no more caused by relaxing than are the disorders which beset a drunkard or an opium-eater, upon refusing to continue in the way of his error, primarily caused by the abandonment of his evil habit, even though the appearance is that he must return to it in order to re-establish his pseudo-equilibrium.

One more cause of trouble, especially in working without a guide, is the habit of going through the form of the exercises without really doing them. The tests needed here have been spoken of before.

Do not separate your way of practising from your way of living, but separate your life entirely from your practice while practising, trying outside of this time always to accomplish the agreement of the two,—that is, live the economy of force that you are practising. You can be just as gay, just as vivacious, but without the fatiguing after-effects.

As you work to gain the ideal equilibrium, if your test comes, do not be staggered nor dismayed. Avoid its increase by at once giving careful consideration to the causes, and dropping them. Keep your life quietly to the form of its usual action, as far as you wisely can. If you have gained even a little appreciation of equilibrium, you will not easily mistake and overdo.

When you find yourself becoming bound to the dismal thought of your test and its terrors, free yourself from it every time, by concentrating upon the weight of your body, or the slowness of the slowest breaths you can draw. Keep yourself truly free, and these feelings of discouragement and all other mental distortions will steadily lose power, until for you they are no more. If they last longer than you think they should, persist in every endeavor, knowing that the after-result, in increased capacity to help yourself and others, will be in exact ratio to your power of persistency without succumbing.

The only way to keep truly free, and therefore ready to profit by the help Nature always has at hand, is to avoid thought of your form of illness as far as possible. The man with indigestion gives the stomach the first place in his mind; he is a mass of detailed and subdued activity, revolving about a monstrous stomach,—his brain, heart, lungs, and other organs, however orderly they may be, are of no consideration, and are slowly made the degraded slaves of himself and his stomach.

The man who does not sleep, worships sleep until all life seems *sleep,* and no life any importance without it. He fixes his mind on not sleeping, rushes for his watch with feverish intensity if a nap does come, to gloat over its brevity or duration, and then wonders that each night brings him no more sleep.

There is nothing more contracting to mind and body than such idol-worship. Neither blood nor nervous fluid can flow as it should.

Let us be sincere in our work, and having gained even one step toward a true equilibrium, hold fast to it, never minding how severely we are tempted.

We see the work of quiet and economy, the lack of strain and of false purpose, in fine old Nature herself; let us constantly try to do our part to make the picture as evident, as clear and distinct, in God's greater creation,—Human Nature.

XVII

THE RATIONAL CARE OF SELF

A WOMAN who had had some weeks of especially difficult work for mind and body, and who had finished it feeling fresh and well, when a friend expressed surprise at her freedom from fatigue, said, with a smiling face: "Oh! but I took great care of myself all through it: I always went to bed early, and rested when it was possible. I was careful to eat only nourishing food, and to have exercise and fresh air when I could get them. You see I knew that the work must be accomplished, and that if I were over-tired I could not do it well." The work, instead of fatiguing, had evidently refreshed her.

If that same woman had insisted, as many have in similar cases, that she had no time to think of herself; or if such care had seemed to her selfish, her work could not have been done as well, she would have ended it tired and jaded, and would have declared to sympathizing friends that it was "impossible to do a work like that without being all tired out," and the sympathizing friends would have agreed and thought her a heroine.

A well-known author, who had to support his wife and family while working for a start in his literary career, had a commercial position that occupied him every day from nine to five. He came home and dined at six, went to bed at seven, slept until three, when he got up, made himself a cup of coffee, and wrote until he breakfasted at eight. He got all the exercise he needed in walking to and from his outside work and was able to keep up this regular routine, with no loss of health, until he could support his family comfortably on what he earned from his pen. Then he returned to ordinary hours.

A brain once roused will take a man much farther than his strength; if this man had come home tired and allowed himself to write far into the night, and then, after a short sleep, had gone to the indispensable earning of his bread and butter, the chances are that his intellectual power would have decreased, until both publishers and author would have felt quite certain that he had no power at all.

The complacent words, "I cannot think of myself," or, "It is out of the question for me to care for myself," or any other of the various forms in which the same idea is expressed, come often from those who are steadily thinking of themselves, and, as a natural consequence, are so blinded that they cannot see the radical difference between unselfish care for one's self, as a means to an end, and the selfish care for one's self which has no other object in view.

The wholesome care is necessary to the best of all good work. The morbid care means steady decay for body and soul.

We should care for our bodies as a violinist cares for his instrument. It is the music that comes from his violin which he has in mind, and he is careful of his instrument because of its musical power. So we, with some sense of the possible power of a healthy body, should be careful to keep it fully supplied with fresh air; to keep it exercised and rested; to supply it with the quality and quantity of nourishment it needs; and to protect it from unnecessary exposure. When, through mistake or for any other reason, our bodies get out of order, instead of dwelling on our discomfort, we should take immediate steps to bring them back to a normal state.

If we learned to do this as a matter of course, as we keep our hands clean, even though we had to be conscious of our bodies for a short time while we were gaining the power, the normal care would lead to a happy unconsciousness. Carlyle says, and very truly, that we are conscious of no part of our bodies until it is out of order, and it certainly follows that the habit of keeping our bodies in order would lead us eventually to a physical freedom which, since our childhood, few of us have known. In the same way we can take care of our minds with a wholesome spirit. We can see to it that they are exercised to apply themselves well, that they are properly diverted, and know how to change, easily, from one kind of work to another. We can be careful not to attempt to sleep directly after severe mental work, but first to refresh our minds by turning our attention into entirely different channels in the way of exercise or amusement.

We must not allow our minds to be over-fatigued any more than our bodies, and we must learn how to keep them in a state of quiet readiness for whatever work or emergency may be before them.

There is also a kind of moral care which is quite in line with the care of the mind and the body, and which is a very material aid to these,—a way of refusing to be irritable, of gaining and maintaining cheerfulness, kindness, and thoughtfulness for others.

It is well known how much the health of any one part of us depends upon all the others. The theme of one of Howells's novels is the steady mental, moral, and physical degeneration of a man from eating a piece of cold mince-pie at midnight, and the sequence of steps by which he is led down is a very natural process. Indeed, how much irritability and unkindness might be traced to chronic indigestion, which originally must have come from some careless disobedience of simple physical laws.

When the stomach is out of order, it needs more than its share of vital force to do its work, and necessarily robs the brain; but when it is in good condition this force may be used for mental work. Then again, when we are in a condition of mental strain or unhealthy concentration, this condition affects our circulation and consumes force that should properly be doing its work elsewhere, and in this way the normal balance of our bodies is disturbed.

The physical and mental degeneration that follows upon moral wrong-doing is too well known to dwell upon. It is self-evident in conspicuous cases, and very real in cases that are too slight to attract general attention. We might almost say that little ways of wrongdoing often produce a worse degeneration, for they are more subtle in their effects, and more difficult to realize, and therefore to eradicate.

The wise care for one's self is simply steering into the currents of law and order,—mentally, morally, and physically. When we are once established in that life and our forces are adjusted to its currents, then we can forget ourselves, but not before: and no one can find these currents of law and order and establish himself in them, unless he is working for some purpose beyond his own health. For a man may be out of order physically, mentally, or morally simply for the want of an aim in life beyond his own personal concerns. No care is to any purpose—indeed, it is injurious—unless we are determined to work for an end which is not only useful in itself, but is cultivating in us a living interest in accomplishment, and leading us on to more usefulness and more accomplishment. The physical, mental, and moral man are all three mutually interdependent, but all the care in the world for each and all of them can only lead to weakness instead of strength, unless they are all three united in a definite purpose of useful life for the benefit of others.

Even a hobby re-acts upon itself and eats up the man who follows it, unless followed to some useful end. A man interested in a hobby for selfish purposes alone first refuses to look at anything outside of his hobby, and later turns his back on everything but his own idea of his hobby. The possible mental contraction which may follow, is almost unlimited, and such contraction affects the whole man.

It is just as certain a law for an individual that what he gives out must have a definite relation to what he takes in, as it is for the best strength of a country that its imports and exports should be in proper balance. Indeed, this law is much more evident in the case of the individual, if we look only a little below the surface. A man can no more expect to live without giving out to others than a shoemaker can expect to earn his bread and butter by making shoes and leaving them piled in a closet.

To be sure, there are many men who are well and happy, and yet, so far as appearances go, are living entirely for themselves, with not only no thought of giving, but a decided unwillingness to give. But their comfort and health are dependent on temporary conditions, and the external well-being they have acquired would vanish, if a serious demand were made upon their characters.

Happy the man or woman who, through illness of body or soul, or through stress of circumstances, is aroused to appreciate the strengthening power of useful work, and develops a wholesome sense of the usefulness and necessity of a rational care of self!

Try to convince a man that it is better on all accounts that he should keep his hands clean and he might answer, "Yes, I appreciate that; but I have never thought of my hands, and to keep them clean would make me conscious of them." Try to convince an unselfishly-selfish or selfishly-unselfish person that the right care for one's self means greater usefulness to others, and you will have a most difficult task. The man with dirty hands is quite right in his answer. To keep his hands clean would make him more conscious of them, but he does not see that, after he had acquired the habit of cleanliness, he would only be conscious of his hands when they were dirty, and that this consciousness could be at any time relieved by soap and water. The selfishly-unselfish person is right: it is most pernicious to care for one's self in a self-centred spirit; and if we cannot get a clear sense of wholesome care of self, it is better not to care at all.

With a perception of the need for such wholesome care, would come a growing realization of the morbidness of all self-centred care, and a clearer, more definite standard of unselfishness. For the self-centred care takes away life, closes the sympathies, and makes useful service obnoxious to us; whereas the wholesome care, with useful service as an end, gives renewed life, an open sympathy, and growing power for further usefulness.

We do not need to study deeply into the laws of health, but simply to obey those we know. This obedience will lead to our knowing more laws and knowing them better, and it will in time become a very simple matter to distinguish the right care from the wrong, and to get a living sense of how power increases with the one, and decreases with the other.

XVIII.

OUR RELATIONS WITH OTHERS

EVERY one will admit that our relations to others should be quiet and clear, in order to give us freedom for our work. Indeed, to make these relations quiet and happy is the special work that some of us have to do. There are laws for health, laws for gaining and keeping normal nerves, laws for honest, kindly action toward others,—but the obedience to all these is a dead obedience, and does not lead to vigorous life, unless accompanied by a hearty love for work and play with those to whom we stand in natural relations,—both young and old. It is with life as it is with art, what we do must be done with love, or it will have no force. Without the living spark of love, we may have the appearance, but never the spirit, of useful work or quiet content. Stagnation is not peace, and there can be no life, and so no living peace, without happy relations with those about us.

The more we realize the practical strength of the law which bids us love our neighbor as ourselves, and the more we act upon it, the more quickly we gain the habit of pleasant, patient friendliness, which sooner or later may beget the same friendliness in return. In this kind of friendly relation there is a savor which so surpasses the unhealthy snap of disagreement, that any one who truly finds it will soon feel the fallacy of the belief that "between friends there must be a little quarrelling, to give spice to friendship."

To be willing that every one should be himself, and work out his salvation in his own way, seems to be the first principle of the working plan drawn from the law of loving your neighbor as yourself. If we drop all selfish resistance to the ways of others, however wrong or ignorant they may be, we are more free to help them to better ways when they turn to us for help. It is in pushing and being pushed that we feel most strain in all human relations.

We wait willingly for the growth of plants, and do not complain, or try in abnormal ways to force them to do what is entirely contrary to the laws of nature; and if we paid more attention to the laws of human nature, we should not stunt the growth of children, relatives, and friends by resisting their efforts,—or their lack of effort,—or by trying to force them into ways that we think must be right for them because we are sure they are right for us.

There is a selfish, restless way of pushing others "for their own good" and straining to "help" them, and there is a selfish, entirely thoughtless way of letting them alone; it is difficult to tell which is the worse, or which does more harm. The first is the attitude of unconscious hypocrisy; the second is that of selfish indifference. It is in letting alone, with a loving readiness to help, that we find strength and peace for ourselves in our relations with others.

All great laws are illustrated most clearly in their simplest forms, and there is no better way to get a sense of really free and wholesome relations with others than from the relations of a mother with her baby. Even healthy reciprocity is there, in all the fulness of its best beginnings, and the results of wholesome, rational, maternal care are evident to the delighted observer in the joyous freedom with which the baby mind develops according to the laws of its own life.

Heidi is a baby not yet a year old, and is left alone a large part of the day. Having no amusements imposed upon her, she has formed the habit of entertaining herself in her own way; she greets you with the most fascinating little gurgles, and laughs up at you when you stop and speak to her as if to say, "How do you do? I am having a *very* happy time!" Five minutes' smiling and being smiled at by her gives a friend who stops to talk "a *very* happy time" too. If you take her up for a little while, she stays quietly and looks at you, then at the trees or at something in the room, then at her own hand. If you say "ah," or "oo," she answers with a vowel too; so the conversation begins and goes on, with jolly little laughter every now and then, and when you give her a gentle kiss and put her down, her good-bye is a very contented one, and her "Thank you; please come again," is quite as plainly understood as if she had said it. You leave her, feeling that you have had a very happy visit with one of your best friends.

Heidi is not officiously interfered with; she has the best of care. When she cries, every means is taken to find the cause of her trouble; and when the trouble is remedied, she stops. She is a dear little friend, and gives and takes, and grows.

Another baby of the same age is Peggy. She is needlessly handled and caressed. She is kissed a hundred times a day with rough affection, which is mistaken for tenderness and love. She is "bounced" up and down and around; and the people about her, who believe themselves her friends and would be heartbroken if she were taken from them, talk at her, and not with her; they make her do "cunning little things," and then laugh and admire; they try over and over to force her to speak words when her little brain is not ready for the effort; and when she is awake, she is almost constantly surrounded by "loving" noise. Peggy is capable of being as good a friend as Heidi, but she is not allowed to be. Her family are so overwhelmed by their own feelings of love and admiration that they really only love themselves in her, for they give her not the slightest opportunity to be herself. The poor baby has sleepless, crying nights, and a little irritating illness hanging about her all the time; the doctor is called, and every one wonders why she should be ill; every one worries about her; but the caressing and noisy affection go on. Although much of the difference between these two babies could probably be accounted for by differences of heredity and temperament, it nevertheless remains true that it is very largely the result of a difference between wise and foolish parents.

The real friendship which her mother gave to Heidi, and which resulted in her happy, placid ways and quickly responsive intelligence, meets with a like response in older children; and reciprocal friendship grows in strength and in pleasure both for child and older friend, as the child grows older. When a child is permitted the freedom of his own individuality, he can show the best in himself. When he is tempted to go wrong, he can be rationally guided in the right way in such a manner that he will accept the guidance as an act of friendship; and to that friendship he will feel bound in honor to be true, because he knows that we, his friends, are obeying the same laws. Of course all this comes to him from no conscious action of his own mind, but from an unconscious, contented recognition of the state of mind of his older friends.

A poor woman, who lived in one room with her husband and two children, said once in a flash of new intelligence, "Now I see: the more I hollers, the more the children hollers; I am not going to holler any more." There are various grades of "hollering;" we "holler" often without a sound, and the child feels it, and "hollers" with many sounds which are distressing to him and to us.

It is primarily true with babies and young children that "if you want to have a friend, you must be a friend." If we want courtesy and kindliness from a child, we must be courteous and kindly to him. Not in outside ways alone,—a child quickly feels the sham of mere superficial attention,— but sincerely, with a living interest.

So should we truly, from our inmost selves, meet a child as if he were of our own age, and as if we were of his age. This sounds like a paradox, but indeed the one proposition is essential to the other. If we meet a child only as if he were of our age, our attitude tends to make him a little prig; if we meet him as if we were as young as he is, his need for maturer influences produces a lack of balance which we must both feet; but if we sincerely meet him as if the exchange of age were mutual, we find common ground and valuable companionship.

This mutual understanding is the basis of all true friendship. Only read, instead of "age," "habit of mind," "character," "state," and we have the whole. It is aiming for reciprocal relations, from the best in us to the best in others, and from the best in others to the best in ourselves. It is the foundation of all that is strengthening, and quiet, and happy, in all human intercourse with young and old.

To gain the friendly habit is more difficult with our contemporaries than it is with children. We have no right to guide older people unless they want to be guided, and they often want to guide us in ways we do not like at all. We have no right to try to change their opinions, unless they ask us for new light; and they often insist upon trying to change ours whether we ask them or not. There is sure to be selfish resistance in us when we complain of it in others, and we must acknowledge it and get free from it before we can give or find the most helpful sympathy.

A healthy letting people alone, and a good wholesome scouring of ourselves, will, if it is to come at all, bring open friendliness. If it is not to come, then the healthy letting people alone should continue, for it is possible to live in the same house with a wilful and trying character, and live at peace, if he is lovingly let alone. If he is unlovingly let alone, the peace will be only on the outside, and must sooner or later give way to storms, or, what is much worse, harden into unforgiving selfishness.

Our influence with others depends primarily upon what we are, and only secondarily upon what we think or upon what we say. It is so with babies and young children, and more so with our older friends. If we honestly feel that there is something for us to learn from another, however wrong or ignorant, in some ways, he may seem, we are not only more able to find and profit by the best in him, but also to give to him in return whatever he may be ready to receive. How little quiet comfort there is in families where useless resistance to one another is habitual! Members of one family often live along together with more or less appearance of good fellowship, but with an inner strain which gives them drawn faces and tired bodies, or else throws them back upon themselves in the enjoyment of their own selfishness; and sometimes there is not even the appearance of good fellowship, but a chronic resistance and disagreement, all for the want of a little sympathy and common sense.

It is the sensitive people that suffer most, and their sensitiveness is deplored by the family and by themselves. If they could only know how great a gift their sensitiveness is! To appreciate this, it must be used to find and feel the good in others, not to make us abnormally alive to real or fancied slights. We must use it to enlarge our sympathies and help us understand the wrong-doing of others enough to point the way, if possible, to better things, not merely to criticise and blame them. Only in such ways can we learn to realize and use the delicate power of sensitiveness. Selfish sensitiveness is a blessing turned to a curse; but the more lovingly sensitive we become to the need of moral freedom in our friends, the Dearer we are led to our own.

There are no human relations that do not illustrate the law which bids me "love my neighbor as myself;" especially clearly is it revealed,—in its breach of observance,—in the comparatively external relations of host and guest in ordinary social life, and in the happiness that can be given and received when it is readily obeyed.

A lady once said, "I go into my bedroom and take note of all the conveniences I have there, and then look about my guest chamber to see that it is equally well and appropriately furnished." She succeeds in her object in the guest chamber if she is the kind of hostess to her guest that she would have her guest be to her; not that her guest's tastes are necessarily her own, but that she knows how to find out what they are and how to satisfy them.

It is often difficult to love our neighbor as ourselves because we do not know how to love ourselves. We are selfish, or stupid, or aggressive with ourselves, or try too hard for what is right and good, instead of trusting with inner confidence and reverence to a power that is above us.

Over-thoughtfulness for others, in little things or great, is oppressive, and as much an enemy to peace, as the lack of any thoughtfulness at all. It is like too much attention to the baby, and comes from the same kind of selfish affection, with—frequently the added motive of wanting to appear disinterested.

One might give pages of examples showing the right and the wrong way in all the varied relations of life, but they would all show that the right way comes from obedience to the law of unselfishness. To obey this law we must respect our neighbor's rights as we respect our own; we must gain and keep the clear and quiet atmosphere that we like to find about our friend; we must shun everything that would interfere with a loving kindliness toward him, as we would have him show the same kindliness toward us. We must know that we and our friends are one, and that, unless a relation is a mutual benefit, it is no true relation at all. But, first of all, we must remember that a true appreciation of the wonderful power of this law comes only with daily, patient working, and waiting for the growth it brings.

In so far as we are truly the friend of one, whether he be baby, child, or grown man,—shall we be truly the friend of all; in so far as we are truly the friend of all, shall we be truly the friend of every one; and, as we find the living peace of this principle, and a greater freedom from selfishness,—whether of affection or dislike,—those who truly belong to us will gravitate to our sides, and we shall gravitate to theirs. Each one of us will understand his own relation to the rest,—whether remote or close,—for in that quiet light it will be seen to rest on intelligible law, which only the fog and confusion of selfishness concealed.

XIX.

THE USE OF THE WILL

IT is not generally recognized that the will can be trained, little by little, by as steadily normal a process as the training of a muscle, and that such training must be through regular daily exercise, and as slow in its effects as the training of a muscle is slow. Perhaps we are unconsciously following, as a race, the law that Froebel has given for the beginnings of individual education, which bids us lead from the "outer to the inner," from the known to the unknown. There is so much more to be done to make methods of muscular training perfect, that we have not yet come to appreciate the necessity for a systematic training of the will. Every individual, however, who recognizes the need of such training and works accordingly, is doing his part to hasten a more intelligent use of the will by humanity in general.

When muscles are trained abnormally their development weakens, instead of strengthening, the whole system. Great muscular strength is often deceptive in the appearance of power that it gives; it often effectually hides, under a strong exterior, a process of degeneration which is going on within, and it is not uncommon for an athlete to die of heart disease or pulmonary consumption.

This is exactly analogous to the frequently deceptive appearance of great strength of will. The will is trained abnormally when it is used only in the direction of personal desire, and the undermining effect upon the character in this case is worse than the weakening result upon the body in the case of abnormal muscular development. A person who is persistently strong in having his own way may be found inconsistently weak when he is thwarted in his own way. This weakness is seldom evident to the general public, because a man with a strong will to accomplish his own ends is quick to detect and hide any appearance of weakness, when he knows that it will interfere with whatever he means to do. The weakness, however, is none the less certainly there, and is often oppressively evident to those from whom he feels that he has nothing to gain.

When the will is truly trained to its best strength, it is trained to obey; not to obey persons or arbitrary ideas, but to obey laws of life which are as fixed and true in their orderly power, as the natural laws which keep the suns and planets in their appointed spheres. There is no one who, after a little serious reflection, may not be quite certain of two or three fixed laws, and as we obey the laws we know, we find that we discover more.

To obey truly we must use our wills to yield as well as to act. Often the greatest strength is gained through persistent yielding, for to yield entirely is the most difficult work a strong will can do, and it is doing the most difficult work that brings the greatest strength.

131

To take a simple example: a small boy with a strong will is troubled with stammering. Every time he stammers it makes him angry, and he pushes and strains and exerts himself with so much effort to speak, that the stammering, in consequence, increases. If he were told to do something active and very painful, and to persist in it until his stammering were cured, he would set his teeth and go through the work like a soldier, so as to be free from the stammering in the shortest possible time. But when he is told that he must relax his body and stop pushing, in order to drop the resistance that causes his trouble, he fights against the idea with all his little might. It is all explained to him, and he understands that it is his only road to smooth speaking; but the inherited tendency to use his will only in resistance is so strong, that at first it seems impossible for him to use it in any other way.

The fact that the will sometimes gains its greatest power by yielding seems such a paradox that it is not strange that it takes us long to realize it. Indeed, the only possible realization of it is through practice.

The example of the little stammering boy is an illustration that applies to many other cases of the same need for giving up resistance.

No matter how actively we need to use our wills, it is often, necessary to drop all self-willed resistance first, before we begin an action, if we want to succeed with the least possible effort and the best result.

When we use the will forcibly to resist or to repress, we are simply straining our nerves and muscles, and are exerting ourselves in a way which must eventually be weakening, not only to them, but to the will itself. We are using the will normally when, without repression or unnecessary effort, we are directing the muscles and nerves in useful work. We want "training and not straining" as much for the will as for the body, and only in that way does the will get its strength.

The world admires a man for the strength of his will if he can control the appearance of anger, whereas the only strength of will that is not spurious is that which controls the anger itself. We have had the habit for so long of living in appearances, that it is only by a slow process that we acquire a strong sense of their frailty and lack of genuine value. In order to bring the will, by training, out of the region of appearances into that of realities, we must learn to find the true causes of weakness and use our wills little by little to remove them. To remove the external effect does no permanent good and produces an apparent strength which only hides an increasing weakness.

Imagine, for instance, a woman with an emotional, excitable nature who is suffering from jealousy; she does not call it jealousy, she calls it "sensitive nerves," and the doctors call it "hysteria." She has severe attacks of "sensitive nerves" or "hysteria" every time her jealousy is excited. It is not uncommon for such persistent emotional strain, with its effect upon the circulation and other functions of the body, to bring on organic disease. In such a case the love of admiration, and the strength of will resulting from that selfish desire, makes her show great fortitude, for which she receives much welcome praise. That is the effect she wants, and in the pose of a wonderful character she finds it easy to produce more fortitude—and so win more admiration.

A will that is strong for the wrong, may—if taken in time—become equally strong for the right. Perversion is not, at first, through lack of will, but through the want of true perception to light the way to its intelligent use.

A man sometimes appears to be without power of will who is only using a strong will in the wrong way, but if he continues in his wrong course long enough, his weakness becomes real.

If a woman who begins her nervous degeneration by indulging herself in jealousy—which is really a gross emotion, however she may refine it in appearance—could be made to see the truth, she would, in many cases, be glad to use her will in the right direction, and would become in reality the beautiful character which her friends believe her to be. This is especially true because this moral and nervous perversion often attacks the finest natures. But when such perversion is allowed to continue, the sufferer's strength is always prominent in external dramatic effects, but disappears oppressively when she is brought face to face with realities.

Many people who are nervous invalids, and many who are not, are constantly weakening themselves and making themselves suffer by using their wills vigorously in every way *but* that which is necessary to their moral freedom: by bearing various unhappy effects with so-called stoicism, or fighting against them with their eyes tight shut to the real cause of their suffering, and so hiding an increasing weakness under an appearance of strength.

A ludicrous and gross example of this misuse of the will may be observed in men or women who follow vigorously and ostentatiously paths of self-sacrifice which they have marked out for themselves, while overlooking entirely places where self-denial is not only needed for their better life, but where it would add greatly to the happiness and comfort of others.

It is curious a such weakness is common with people who are apparently very intelligent; and parallel with this are cases of men who are remarkably strong in the line of their own immediate careers, and proportionately weak in every other phase of their lives. We very seldom find a soldier, or a man who is powerful in politics, who can answer in every principle and action of his life to Wordsworth's "Character of the Happy Warrior."

Absurd as futile self-sacrifice seems, it is not less well balanced than the selfish fortitude of a jealous woman or than the apparent strength of a man who can only work forcibly for selfish ends. The wisest use of the will can only grow with the decrease of self-indulgence.

"Nervous" women are very effective examples of the perversion of a strong will. There are women who will work themselves into an illness and seem hopelessly weak when they are not having their own way, who would feel quite able to give dinner parties at which they could be prominent in whatever role they might prefer, and would forget their supposed weakness with astonishing rapidity. When things do not go to please such women, they are weak and ill; when they stand out among their friends according to their own ideal of themselves and are sufficiently flattered, they enter into work which is far beyond their actual strength, and sooner or later break down only to be built up on another false basis.

This strong will turned the wrong way is called "hysteria," or "neurasthenia," or "degeneracy." It may be one of these or all three, *in its effect,* but the training of the will to overcome the cause, which is always to be found in some kind of selfishness, would cure the hysteric, give the neurasthenic more wholesome nerves, and start the degenerate on a course of regeneration. At times it would hardly surprise us to hear that a child with a stomach-ache crying for more candy was being treated for "hysteria" and studied as a "degenerate." Degenerate he certainly is, but only until he can be taught to deny himself candy when it is not good for him, with quiet and content.

There are many petty self-indulgences which, if continually practised, can do great and irreparable harm in undermining the will. Every man or woman knows his own little weaknesses best, but that which leads to the greatest harm is the excuse, "It is my temperament; if I were not tardy, or irritable, or untidy,"—or whatever it may be,—"I would not be myself." Our temperament is given us as a servant, not as a master; and when we discover that an inherited perversion of temperament can be trained to its opposite good, and train it so, we do it not at a loss of individuality, but at a great gain. This excuse of "temperament" is often given as a reason for not yielding.

The family will is dwelt upon with a pride which effectually prevents it from keeping its best strength, and blinds the members of the family to the weakness that is sure to come, sooner or later, as a result of the misuse of the inheritance of which they are so proud.

If we train our wills to be passive or active, as the need may be, in little things, that prepares us for whatever great work may be before us. Just as in the training of a muscle, the daily gentle exercise prepares it to lift a great weight.

Whether in little ways or in great ways, it is stupid and useless to expect to gain real strength, unless we are working in obedience to the laws that govern its development. We have a faculty for distinguishing order from disorder and harmony from discord, which grows in delicacy and strength as we use it, and we can only use it through refusing disorder and choosing order. As our perception grows, we choose more wisely, and as we choose more wisely, our perception grows. But our perceptions must work in causes, not at all in effects, except as they lead us to a knowledge of causes. We must, above all, train our wills as a means of useful work. It is impossible to perfect ourselves for the sake of ourselves.

It is a happy thing to have been taught the right use of the will as a child, but those of us who have not been so taught, can be our own fathers and our own mothers, and we must be content with a slow growth. We are like babies learning to walk. The baby tries day after day, and does not feel any strain, or wake in the morning with a distressing sense of "Oh! I must practise walking to-day. When shall I have finished learning?" He works away, time after time falling down and picking himself up, and some one day finally walks, without thinking about it any more. So we, in the training of our wills, need to work patiently day by day; if we fall, we must pick ourselves up and go on, and just as the laws of balance guide the baby, so the laws of life will carry us.

When the baby has succeeded in walking, he is not elated at his new power, but uses it quietly and naturally to accomplish his ends. We cannot realize too strongly that any elation or personal pride on our part in a better use of the will, not only obstructs its growth, but is directly and immediately weakening.

A quiet, intelligent use of the will is at the root of all character; and unselfish, well-balanced character, with the insight which it develops, will lead us to well-balanced nerves.

SUMMING UP

TO sum it all up, the nerves are conductors for impression and expression. As channels, they should be as free as Emerson's "smooth hollow tube," for transmission from without in, and from within out. Thus the impressions will be clear, and the expressions powerful.

The perversions in the way of allowing to the nerves the clear conducting power which Nature would give them are, so far as the body is concerned, unnecessary fatigue and strain caused by not resting entirely when the times come for rest, and by working with more than the amount of force needed to accomplish our ends,—thus defying the natural laws of equilibrium and economy. Not only in the ways mentioned do we defy these most powerful laws, but, because of carelessness in nourishment and want of normal exercise out of doors, we make the establishment of such equilibrium impossible.

The nerves can never be open channels while the body wants either proper nourishment, the stimulus that comes from open air exercise, perfect rest, or true economy of force in running the human machine.

The physical training should be a steady shunning of personal perversions until the nervous system is in a natural state, and the muscles work in direct obedience to the will with the exquisite co-ordination which is natural to them.

The same equilibrium must be found in the use of the mind. Rest must be complete when taken, and must balance the effort in work,—rest meaning often some form of recreation as well as the passive rest of steep. Economy of effort should be gained through normal concentration,—that is, the power of erasing all previous impressions and allowing a subject to hold and carry us, by dropping every thought or effort that interferes with it, in muscle, nerve, and mind. The nerves of the senses must be kept clear through this same ability to drop all previous impressions.

First in importance, and running all through the previous training, is the use of the will, from which all these servants, mental and physical, receive their orders,—true or otherwise as the will itself obeys natural and spiritual laws in giving them. The perversions in the will to be shunned are misuse of muscles by want of economy in force and power of direction; abuse of the nervous system by unwisely dwelling upon pain and illness beyond the necessary care for the relief of either, or by allowing sham emotions, irritability, and all other causes of nervous distemper to overcome us.

The remedy for this is to make a peaceful state possible through a normal training of the physique; to realize and follow a wholesome life in all its phases; to recognize daily more fully through obedience the great laws of life by which we must be governed, as certainly as an engineer must obey the laws of mechanics if he wants to build a bridge, that will stand, as certainly as a musician must obey the laws of harmony if he would write good music, as surely as a painter must obey the laws of perspective and of color if he wishes to illuminate Nature by means of his art.

No matter what our work in life, whether scientific, artistic, or domestic, it is the same body through which the power is transmitted; and the same freedom in the conductors for impression and expression is needed, to whatever end the power may be moved, from the most simple action to the highest scientific or artistic attainment.

The quality of power differs greatly; the results are widely different, but the laws of transmission are the same. So wonderful is the unity of life and its laws!

140

THE END

www.ingramcontent.com/pod-product-compliance
Lightning Source LLC
Chambersburg PA
CBHW070251190526

45169CB00001B/371